Dark Psychology

And

Manipulation

How to Stop Being Manipulated, the Secrets and
the Art of Reading People.

Psychology of Persuasion, of Narcissist and
Machiavellian Human Behavior.

Winning Influence.

By Ray Manson

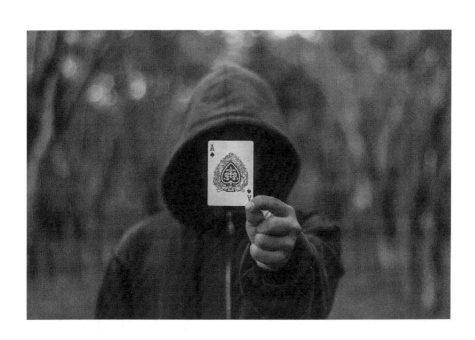

Table of Contents

Introduction 9

Chapter 1: The Darkness of Dark Psychology 13

Chapter 2: The Dark Traits 37

Chapter 3: The Machiavellian 50

Chapter 4: The Narcissist 57

Chapter 5: The Psychopath 84

Chapter 6: The Everyday Sadist 113

Chapter 7: Dark Techniques 124

Chapter 8: Manipulation 128

Chapter 9: Brainwashing/Mind Control 144

Chapter 10: Seduction 150

Chapter 11: The Dark End 156

This Book is provided with the sole purpose of providing relevant information on a specific topic for which every reasonable effort has been made to ensure that it is both accurate and reasonable. Nevertheless, by purchasing this Book you consent to the fact that the author, as well as the publisher, are in no way experts on the topics contained herein, regardless of any claims as such that may be made within. As such, any suggestions or recommendations that are made within are done so purely for entertainment value. It is recommended that you always consult a professional prior to undertaking any of the advice or techniques discussed within.

This is a legally binding declaration that is considered both valid and fair by both the Committee of Publishers Association and the American Bar Association and should be considered as legally binding within the United States.

The reproduction, transmission, and duplication of any of the content found herein, including any specific or extended information will be done as an illegal act regardless of the end form the information ultimately takes. This includes copied versions of the work both physical, digital and audio unless express consent of the Publisher is provided beforehand. Any additional rights reserved.

Furthermore, the information that can be found within the pages described forthwith shall be considered both accurate and truthful when it comes to the recounting of facts. As such, any use, correct or incorrect, of the provided information will render the Publisher free of responsibility as to the actions taken outside of their direct purview. Regardless, there are zero scenarios where the original author or the Publisher can be deemed liable in any fashion for any damages or hardships that may result from any of the information discussed herein.

Additionally, the information in the following pages is intended only for informational purposes and should thus be thought of as universal. As befitting its nature, it is presented without assurance regarding its prolonged validity or interim quality. Trademarks that are mentioned are done without written consent and can in no way be considered an endorsement from the trademark holder.

Introduction

There is a capacity of virtue in us, and there is a capacity of vice to make your blood creep.

Ralph Waldo Emerson, "Nature"

If psychology is the study of the mind and human behavior, with the goal largely being that it helps people achieve insights into their own actions in order to give them a better understanding of themselves and others, there's a kind of built-in assumption, even on the part of those who have no real idea what psychology's all about or what exactly it is psychologists do, that psychology is more about the science of what is wrong in people than what is right. (In the same way most people turn to doctors for help with what's ailing them than for a pat on the shoulder for having cared for themselves so well that they've never even needed a doctor.) Psychologists, then, like doctors, we look to for explanations more about what's *not* right about us, or what's *not* right about others, than for what *is* right.

So while it may seem redundant to take the field of psychology one step further, into the world of dark psychology—isn't psychology itself pretty dark? Aren't most of the things that psychologists study and deal with bad enough—schizophrenia, obsessive-compulsive disorder, depression, manias of all kinds, phobias of all kinds, fear, anxiety? What could be darker than psychology itself? Why *dark* psychology? Have people in the past 10 years, 20 years, in the past century, become worse than they were at any other time in history? Did we never have narcissists before? Or sadists? Or charismatic leaders and abusive spouses?

The answer, which is obvious, is no. History is chockfull of sadists and con men, pedophiles and Machiavellis. Niccolo Machiavelli may have been the first to write a book exclusively and explicitly about the Machiavelli type—the unscrupulous politicians he saw all around him in late-15th and early-16th century Italy, as typified in his 1513 book, *The Prince.* But these types, these two-faced schemers with little to no morals, no empathy for others, and whose laserlike focus on their own gain is, well, what we've come to call Machiavellian—they've also been around since time immemorial.

What's new, what dark psychology is getting at, what it's dealing with, the people and traits with which it's most concerned—*dark* psychology may come off to some as a little redundant. But where psychology tries to rationalize what drives people to do the things they do and explain why it is people behave the way they behave, dark psychology says, No.

There are people out there, and they are very dangerous people, who do things that are beyond explanation, beyond reason, whose actions cannot be explained. And the best the rest of us can do, psychologists and psychiatrists and therapists and everyone else, is to keep trying to figure out why, even though there may be no good reason. But with the idea that we do so in order to better understand how to deal with these dark forces and dark individuals. The closer we can get to an understanding, if not exactly an explanation of why these people do the things they do, and what drives them to commit such acts, the better the chance of helping them. And helping ourselves.

Chapter 1: The Darkness of Dark Psychology

No one becomes depraved all at once.

Juvenal, *Satires*

The great epochs of our lives are the occasions when we gain the courage to rebaptize our evil qualities as our best qualities

Friedrich Nietzsche, *Beyond Good and Evil*

Dark Psychology really came to light in 2002, when Delroy Paulhus , a personality psychology researcher and professor of psychology at the University of British Columbia, and Kevin Williams, a research scientist with the Educational Testing Service, published their paper, "The Dark Triad of Personality: Narcissism, Machiavellianism, and Psychopathy." In it the two laid out the personality traits for what they called the Dark Triad. These traits were: Narcissism (entitled self-importance), Machiavellianism (the manipulation of others for one's own gains), and Psychopathy (an antisocial individual completely lacking in empathy or remorse). Since that paper came out, thousands of other papers on the Dark Triad (and Dark Psychology) have appeared, with over 1,700 coming out in 2018 alone. And that's not counting the many thousands of articles, essays, opinion pieces, blogs—and websites devoted almost exclusively to the Dark Triad—that have also appeared in the past 10 years.

What Paulhus and Williams laid out in that groundbreaking paper (in which they sampled 245 university students) was the idea that these three traits tend to exist along a spectrum (not unlike Asperger's or Autism), that the personalities of the Dark Triad move in and out of each other, even though they are otherwise distinct from one another, and rarely are all three present in one person (or rarely all three together to the extreme that that person would then qualify as having a mental disorder), and that all of us are at least a little bit narcissistic, a little bit Machiavellian, and a little bit psychopathic.

These socially aversive traits have been around for centuries. And since Paulhus and Williams' paper came out, other researchers, particularly evolutionary biologists, have been questioning the Darwinian roots of these traits: are these personality traits somehow biologically necessary to the reproduction of the species? Are they genetically rewarded? What is the value of these traits to the prolongation of humans? And on a grander scale, given that these three traits are so seemingly loathsome and undesirable, why are they a part of us? What do they contribute to the overall balance and harmony of nature? Of human nature? How do they factor in biologically and evolutionarily, and why do they seem to survive and thrive not only in individuals but in societies? Do they preserve a balance between a civilized world and anarchy? Or are they leading us down the path to collective suicide?

The Dark Side of Genetics

As Lyall Watson put it in his book *Dark Nature: A Natural History of Evil*, Darwin, creator of the concept of survival of the fittest, viewed morality as humankind's cure for inner conflicts. He predicted that if any other species aside from our own were to secure intellectual abilities that they would in time also develop a conscience, a set of morals. Watson agreed with Darwin's theory, and felt that whatever morals evolved in us, they would only become that much stronger alongside knowing what was immoral.

Watson, though, trained as a botanist, zoologist, and ethologist (and, interestingly enough, originator of the hypothetical Hundredth Monkey Effect), and ever the reluctant Darwinian here in his study of evil and its utility, looks at evil from the biological perspective. And so defines evil as anything that upsets the integrity of an ecological environment, anything that discombobulates diversity, abundance or communications. And while Watson the biologist can understand why almost every species, from a cellular level, feels compelled to kill off any stranger that comes into its midst, and can appreciate infanticide among lions and birds, he is stumped—as are most of us—by the Pol Pots and the Ted Bundys of the world.

His ultimate conclusion was rather desultory: the world is immoral though we are not. Natural selection is unavoidable, and devoid of any feeling. Genetic evolution, then, favors a kind of selfish behavior—on the individual level and on the bigger scale of humans as a species. As Watson puts it: It's OK and even necessary for our reproduction to be nice to people, but only to those in our bloodline. To those outside our bloodline, don't trust them, don't feel obligated to be nice to them. And lie, cheat, and steal whenever you can. Our genes require this sort of behavior if we are to survive. The happiness of everyone else be damned.

Short-Term Success

In 2009, another seminal study in the field of the Dark Triad came out. In this one, "The Dark Triad: Facilitating a Short-Term Mating Strategy in Men," psychologist Peter Jonason and colleagues looked at the Dark Triad through the lens of evolution, asking whether or not these dark traits might give individuals an advantage in the world. In their introduction they state the reasons behind their paper have to do with their suspicion that Dark Triad traits don't just pop out of the blue within people but they have a kind of evolutionary advantage. People seek out those with Dark Traits because those Dark Trait carriers have a greater chance to reproduce. Never mind that these Dark Traits tend to be have dark results, for individuals and society, they're beneficial in the long run. Psychopaths of the subclinical type tend not to be neurotic or anxietal, which gives these characters advantages when it comes to hooking up. Narcissists, too, who are largely out for themselves, and Machiavellians, who are experts at working other people, usually excel in one-night stands and short relationships. Anything long-term usually doesn't pan out, even though they tend to leave others damaged in their wake, what do these types care. They got what they wanted. And they don't want anything beyond their short-term needs.

In other words, these Dark Personality Alpha Joe types get ahead of everyone else at work, get laid more often (and with women who seem to attract, and seem most attracted to, the alpha males), and otherwise "succeed" in life.

Again, as with Paulhus and Williams' paper, this study not only gave the Dark Triad that much more credibility but the media, especially the media covering the industries of business and finance, embraced it. Practically wholeheartedly. While plenty of folks lamented the findings and assertions put forth by Jonason, decrying the idea that society tends to reward psychopaths and narcissists, many a ruthless CEO and more than a few pickup artists felt both vindicated and emboldened. If the absence of anxiety and neuroticism led to bedding more women (whether or not all these notches on the bedpost led to more babies, i.e, whether or not it led to the genetic reproduction and continuation of that psychopath's, that narcissist's, that Machiavellian's DNA), over and above the Joe Schmoes of the world vainly trying to woo women with roses and understanding and the Old World values of a good, honest man, then it made just as much sense that having a narcissistic knack for self-aggrandizement and the charisma of a psychopath would give Manny Machiavelli a leg up in the hypercompetitive worlds of business and politics.

The Dirty Dozen

Then, in 2010, Jonason emerged again, this time with a 12-item questionnaire he and his colleague Gregory Webster of the University of Florida cynically named the Dirty Dozen. Devised with the goal of providing other researchers with a cleaner, clearer and cheaper way to measure the latent constructs of the Dark Triad, the Dirty Dozen is a Cliff's Notes mashup of the Minnesota Multiphasic Personality Inventory and the Wonderlic test, boiled down to 12 statements. The higher the score, the higher one's Dark Triad tendencies.

Ruthless, Counterproductive, Toxic

Two years later, in 2012, Ernest O'Boyle and colleagues at the School of Business and Economics at Longwood University in Virginia released the results of a meta-analysis of studies of the Dark Triad. Wanting to know what sorts of impact individuals with these Dark traits were having in the workplace, they discovered that Machiavellians and Psychopaths had a negative effect on the workplace and on coworkers—not a positive one. Job performance went down.

A few years later, in an update on how things were going in the world of Dark Triad research (since Pauhlus and Williams' groundbreaking paper, there'd been dozens of studies and over 350 scholarly citations), Adrian Furnham, a professor of psychology at University College London, along with Paulhus himself and a fellow UC London psychology colleague, released "The Dark Triad of Personality: A 10-Year Review." Almost anticlimactic in its principle finding, the three psychologists agreed that people of the Dark Triad stepped all over others in their desire to climb the corporate ladder. And while these types correlated positively with each other, each of the three Dark Triad traits were nevertheless unique: Machiavellians appear more likely to plagiarize essays and avoid risky bets; Narcissists are often more aggressive after any sort of threat to their ego; and Psychopaths torment others and not only entertain more revenge fantasies but are more likely to follow through on them. Worse, the authors claimed that any one of these Dark Personality types made for horrible bosses, so bad that they were ultimately bad for business.

What's Bad May Be Good—for Business

But the tide against the Dark Triad soon began to shift. What were once regarded as malignant traits suddenly became useful if not downright admirable. In the 2015 study, "Do Bad Guys Get Ahead or Fall Behind? Relationships of the Dark Triad of Personality With Objective and Subjective Career Success," published by three Swiss psychologists, the authors decided that having these Dark characters in the workplace maybe wasn't so bad after all. Narcissists made more money (for themselves and on occasion for their company), Machiavellians made for effective leaders and loved their jobs, only the Psychopaths seemed to have and create a hard time.

In other words: score another one for the bad guys. Who were quickly turning into . . . not-so-bad guys. Or bad guys who happen to be more successful than good guys. Narcissism seemed to correlate with higher salaries, Machiavellianism led individuals further up the career ladder, and psychopaths seemed to outnumber non-psychopaths in leadership positions in the business world.

These dark traits, this Dark Triad of Dark Psychology, the more people seemed to study it, the more people seemed to admire it and embrace it. And not grudgingly but as traits to aspire to. As practicing clinical psychologist Noam Shpancer put it in a 2017 story for *Psychology Today*, echoing the cynicism of Lyall Watson, the world, especially the business world, can be a mean place. Better to be mean back to it, and to the other mean people out there. And if that means mirroring the behaviors of those in the Dark Triad, so be it. Still, as much as he "praised" the qualities of these Dark Personality types, he did allow for all the trouble they cause: lying, cheating, bullying.

If you're a member of the Dark Triad, such backhanded compliments like Shpancer's come off as so much jealousy, as yet another good guy whining about how he can't get ahead in life, moaning on and on about women always pining after bad boys. Shpancer's caveat here smacks of the usual Judeo-Christian argument of last resort: Sure, you're rich, you have the most beautiful wife in the state, you've crushed all your business rivals, you do pretty much whatever (and whoever) you want, but are you happy? Are you really and truly happy? Don't you know that it pays, in the end, on your deathbed, when you're at the pearly gates, to have been kind to people? To have been compassionate and generous—not selfish and mean-spirited? Even if it is in your Darwinian genes to have lived that way. This Dark Triad you lived your life by, that didn't really bring you happiness, and it probably wasn't the only reason you were so "successful."

By the end of his Dark Triad article, Shpancer sounds like the parent of an underachieving millennial, grudgingly accepting all the accomplishments of the Dark Triad types, while adding that, even so, they don't make for great supervisors, lovers, or bosom buddies.

Who's More Interesting?

Paulhus, for one, can't get enough of them. Perhaps not in real life, but certainly as subjects for continuous study. In his 2014 paper, "Toward a Taxonomy of Dark Personalities," he's practically giddy. His appreciation for all the "good" in them is understandable. After all, he's essentially made his career out of studying them. (So to want them locked up and put away, evolutionarily, would deprive him of a source of study. Despite all the evil inside them, and the havoc they tend to wreak, Paulhus, like many researchers out there, and plenty of laypeople who want to know more about these Dark Traits and how they may be of use to their lives (their love lives, their careers), kinda likes them.

So just who are these Dark Personality types? In Dark Triad (or Tetrad) terms, what is a Machiavellian? A Narcissist? A Psychopath? An everyday Sadist? According to Paulhus and others, all four score high, and essentially meet, on callousness (a lack of empathy for other people). Narcissists have no concern for the well-being of those who stand in the way of what they want. Machiavellians proceed cunningly, always looking two or three steps ahead of their competitors and keeping an eye on whoever might be monitoring them. And Psychopaths just take whatever they want from whoever's closest. And the Everyday Sadist? They just like to watch others hurt, and it's all the more delectable when they're the ones who bring the pain.

As a group, these characters are self-centered and socially offensive. However, they also tend to be extroverts, outgoing and sociable, charming, and often make very good first impressions. And Paulhus, again editorializing to the point of giddiness over his enthusiasm for these Dark personality types, states in his "Taxonomy" that these folks have a knack for shifting gears; if the situation or the context changes, they change with it. How adaptive are they? People often find Narcissists alluring, but only for so long—as in, say, as long as it takes to make that good first impression in a job interview or a first date. But spending any time around them beyond those first impressions and they begin to wear. As for Psychopaths, given the right context, say, a street gang, they can flourish. And the Everyday Sadist would do well in a profession that involves enforcement or inflicting punishment.

And this is where Paulhus' biases lean in favor of the Dark Triad types. When he asks, rhetorically, whether hiring any of these Tetrad types would be worth the risk, his response is, Why not? They're not boring. And they can probably increase your earnings. And they likely won't be standing around at the Christmas party with a lampshade over their heads.
So, yes. Charming—but with no regard for the feelings of others.

Clinical Vs. Subclinical

Which leads Paulhus to probably the most important question: Are these Dark Personalities clinically disturbed? Or are they subclinical conditions? In his opinion, and the opinions of other psychologists, these Dark Traits, while they can be admittedly pushy, deceitful, kinda scary, unless you're keen on factoring in their scores for hostility, no, they don't quality as more than subclinical.

It's a distinction that, from the outside, from the layperson's perspective, from the point of view of someone who's having to deal with a Machiavellian, a Psychopath, a Narcissist, hardly matters. These Dark Personality types are putting other people through Hell, and trying to explain to them the difference between a clinical Psychopath and a subclinical Psychopath— do the people on the receiving end of these Dark behaviors really care? Most just want to get away from their tormentor. It doesn't help that one may be short-term (subclinical) and the other longer-lasting (clinical). Or that a clinical Psychopath is—better at what he does than the subclinical Psychopath? Has been at it longer? Might have a harder time changing his ways?

In their book, *Almost a Psychopath: Do I (or Does Someone I Know) Have a Problem with Manipulation and Lack of Empathy?*, Ronald Shouten and James Silver tried to explain the difference between the full-on clinical Psychopath and the kinda-sorta subclinical psychopath. Their idea of a full-on member of the Dark Tetrad versus the kinda-sorta Dark Triad player, well, there's not much of a tangible difference.

The main difference for them has to do with how long these Dark Personality types, the clinical ones, last in the workplace or in a relationship. In their opinion, they don't last long. and they tend not to want to stick around anyway. The other distinction, according to Shouten and Silver, and many other psychologists and psychiatrists, comes down to grandiosity. Or the level of grandiosity. And perhaps it's about sustainability as well. The kinda-sorta psychopaths, it seems, don't have the stamina of the true clinical psychopath. Or the kinda-sorta psychopath has only two of the three necessary traits exhibited by the true psychopath. If this strikes many as picayune and beside the point—I'm being tortured here every day by this awful CEO who thinks he's the Master of the Universe!—it's this type of hairsplitting that, when you're the person who's under the thumb of a Narcissist, a Machiavellian, a Psychopath, does it really matter if they're only a kinda-sorta Machiavellian or a kinda-sorta Narcissist?

Predators without Purpose

As news of the Dark Triad spread, and people outside and even inside the world of psychology began to realize just how destructive these Dark Forces could be, the distinctions between almost and for real didn't matter as much as the actual physical, psychological, emotional, and spiritual damage being done by these Dark personality types. Dark Psychology as a term in and of itself became so all-encompassing and seductive, it could account for practically anything and everything that had previously been described as just plain evil.

Such has been the allure of Dark Psychology to New York state-licensed psychologist Michael Nuccitelli. A graduate of Chicago's Adler University (and hence, a proponent of the university's namesake, Alfred Adler, a colleague of Freud's, founder of the school of individual psychology, and the originator of the idea of the inferiority complex—significant in relation to the Dark Triad because of how it addresses the matter of individual self-esteem, and the danger of a person with an inferiority complex being that she might seek to overcome that feeling by turning egocentric, power-hungry, and aggressive), Nuccitelli so fully bought into everything that Dark Psychology represented that by 2009 he'd not only incorporated it into his practice, but had made it his life's calling. Up until that time Nuccitelli had been working in the field of forensic psychology, conducting evaluations and consultations for attorneys and the courts. But after seeing the nefarious ooze of Dark Psychology and how it had wormed its way into the lives of so many people, he turned his attention to the study of the Dark Personality types out there in cyberspace.

For Nuccitelli, Dark Psychology comes down to predators (the Dark Actors) and the prey—the rest of us. These Dark Actors prey on others, and no matter what type they are, they're either criminals or deviants or both. He has made it his calling to figure out why they do what they do, and to try to stop them.

Dark Individuals with Dark Thoughts Moving Along a Dark Continuum . . .

And where others often talk about Dark Psychology as existing along a spectrum, as first proposed by Paulhus and Williams, and to which many other researchers and psychologists readily admit is likely the case for most if not all of us, Nuccitelli puts that in, well, even darker terms: Everyone has Dark Thoughts. Unlike the rest of us, though, these Dark Individuals follow through on their fantasies and desires. And they do so with no discernible reason. They just do it because they can. And rather than addressing it as a spectrum, he has named this range the Dark Continuum. Dark Psychology is a fancier term for the dark side.

It is the individual who is not interested in his fellow men who has the greatest difficulties in life and provides the greatest injury to others. It is from among such individuals that all human failures spring.

Alfred Adler, *What Life Could Mean to You*

. . . and into the Dark Singularity

Not surprisingly, Nuccitelli looks at the Dark Triad from, and bases his theories of Dark Psychology on, a largely Adlerian perspective. It was Adler's belief that all human behavior is purposive; everything we think, feel, do has a purpose, and pretty much nothing we set into motion happens randomly (not that random things can't happen *to* us, just that whatever we do, we do with intent). When individuals are brought up in an environment that makes them feel accepted, like they belong, that gives them a purpose, they turn out well. But if these individuals feel like their environment's not welcoming,

But if these developing individuals see others as out to harm them, or trying to manipulate them, Darkness beckons. Which becomes all the more difficult to resist when it's inside all of us anyway. And if we're saddled with any trace of an inferiority complex, the concept that Adler came up with, hello Darkness. Evil for these neglected types becomes their calling. The narcissistic psychopath, for one, serves as the perfect example of Adler's inferiority complex gone haywire.

All in all, Nuccitelli seems to have little confidence in humans. Even while trying to couch our Dark Psychology in Darwinian terms, he sounds like Tommy Lee Jones' character trying to explain the inexplicably cold murderous hitman played by Javier Bardem in *No Country for Old Men*. We all have bad thoughts. We all entertain the idea of taking out our violent fantasies on others. The Dark Actors, unlike most of us, act out these nightmares.

Nuccitelli, then, sees only evil in Dark Psychology. Evil people, evil acts, evil that's pointing to what he calls a Dark Singularity—a kind of evil version of the internet singularity, wherein a Dark Individual's appetite becomes, equivalent to the technological singularity uncontrollable, unquenchable, unattainable, resulting in nothing but death and destruction. He sees the internet, and pretty much everything technological, as fitting hand in glove with the goals of the Dark Individual.

Luckily, these Dark Individuals won't ever band together, becoming an army or a race of autonomous Terminators or cybernetically enhanced serial killers. These Dark Individuals will never emerge as an army under someone else's control, either, doing the bidding of the Ultimate Dark Individual (at least, there's been no talk yet, from Nuccitelli or Jonas or anyone else, predicting such a person or scenario), mostly because they're too focused on themselves and *only* on themselves.

Nevertheless, they are a new breed. And we seem to be producing more and more Dark Individuals. Especially when such traits are praised and valued without proper qualification. Especially, too, that these individuals seem to have found a home in the digital spheres.

Dark Shadows

The shadow is a living part of the personality and therefore wants to live with it in some form. It cannot be argued out of existence or rationalized into harmlessness.

Carl Jung, *The Archetypes*
and the Collective Unconscious

As despairing as people like Nuccitelli appear to be, there are positives to this Dark Psychology (even while there are also aspects to this darkness that are downright terrifying). Paulhus and Jonason have obviously seen something redeeming if not actually helpful to these dark traits. But the person most responsible for awakening others to the benefits of our darker proclivities would have to be Carl Jung, the early 20th century founder of analytical psychology (and onetime colleague, like Adler, of Sigmund Freud).

It was Jung who first gave name to this unconscious, id-like side to our personality. It's the unknown part of the self, the side the ego almost refuses to identify. It's the flipside to our outward self, our persona. Hence, it's tendency to remain in our psychological shadows. And because most people are ignorant of it, fearful of it because it seems to carry our least desirable aspects, most people tend to regard it as negative.

Jung, though, saw it as necessary, vital even to our overall mental health. But only if we acknowledged it, dealt with it, brought it out (at least occasionally) into the light. we're all light and dark, good and evil. But the more we tamp down that shadowy part of ourselves, it doesn't go away. It just rears its black head in other ways.

Jung's point in naming the shadow was to first bring it to everyone's awareness, and then from there, not to shame people into the realization that they have a dark side, but to encourage people to embrace their shadow side in order to become a fully integrated, healthy human being. Recognizing our shadow and dealing with it allows us to become whole. Not just whole but better, more creative, more open to others. Confronting this part of ourselves not only "completed" us but had the potential to open us up to larger, more creative, more aspirational selves. It's the shadow that many others later saw as the source of our true creativity. Or our true potential.

After citing Richard Nixon as one of the worst versions of someone who embraced and gave to the world the most inauthentic versions of their repressed shadow, international best-selling author Robert Greene, in *The Laws of Human Nature* (his 2018 follow-up to *The 48 Laws of Power* and *The*

Art of Seduction), then lists some of the best examples of those who epitomize Jung's fully integrated human: Winston Churchill, Abraham Lincoln, Albert Einstein, Charlie Chaplin, and Jacqueline Kennedy-Onassis. These are people who saw the positives in their shadow side. And let that shadow out to play.

The forces that get in the way of our true selves are mainly our parents, and later, the rest of society. Growing up, that shadow side could express itself. But as we aged, our parents, teachers, even our friends convinced us to hold back our shadow. Society functions better when we're not all out there letting our shadows run free. So we caved in. Much to our own loss and regret.

It's less heady, less psychoanalytical version of what Jung and others after him laid out as the reasons behind so many of us having repressed this darker aspect of our personalities. Greene is no less a champion, though, of all the benefits to be gained by embracing one's Shadow. Embrace it, he implores his readers. That's where all the good stuff is. Even the scariest parts—the ones that others characterize as criminal. That's OK. Entertaining the fantasy of beating up that tailgater behind you, or telling your boss to go F himself, that's fine. Just don't do it in real life.

Someone I loved once gave me a box full of darkness. It took me years to understand that this too, was a gift.

Mary Oliver

As if we might not be convinced enough, Greene then brings out the poster boy for the Shadow—the Shadow at its absolute best, the Shadow at its most naked, in the form of late CEO and co-founder of Apple, Steve Jobs. Greene, like many, idolizes Jobs. And epitomizes how we could be, all of us, if we just had the courage he had, if we just had his balls, his chutzpah, to give our dark side just enough leash so that it could run freely, only never off the leash so as to be out of our control. He respected his shadow. He kept it close by. He understood that his shadow not only allowed him to tap into and express his creativity, it also gave him a huge advantage over his peers in the high-tech industry. Jobs had an edge. And that edge sometimes came with a price. But look at the payoff. Jobs changed the global culture. Would that have happened if he had listened to everyone else? If he'd kept his shadow in the closet like the rest of us? Probably not, says Greene.

As we'll see later on, in light of what Dark Psychology has given us, Steve Jobs has come to be seen as borderline. To some, not all that different from the most Machiavellian, most narcissistic, most psychopathic of leaders. These off-putting qualities excused only by his genius and for the products he gave the world.

Jobs is also enlightening for what Dark Psychology is and how it differs from the more pathological, the more clinical definitions of a sadist, a psychopath, a narcissist. What often separates the men from the boys, so to speak, the Dark Personalities from the Darkest of Personalities, is often a matter of degree, scale, style, and intent.

Chapter 2: The Dark Traits

This longing to commit a madness stays with us throughout our lives. Who has not, when standing with someone by an abyss or high up on a tower, had a sudden impulse to push the other over? And how is it that we hurt those we love although we know that remorse will follow? Our whole being is nothing but a fight against the dark forces within ourselves. To live is to war with trolls in heart and soul.

Playwright Henrik Ibsen

Since the introduction of the Dark Triad in 2002, the triad itself has remained surprisingly stable. There's the Machiavellian, the Narcissist, and the Psychopath (although, technically, the last two would be classified by psychologists as the subclinical Narcissist and the subclinical Psychopath). And while there might be some quibbling about the exact characteristics of each of these dark traits, they, too, have remained pretty consistent. But when Delroy Paulhus expanded the traits from three to four, from triad to tetrad, with his "Taxonomy" paper in 2014, opening the door to the

Everyday Sadist, the traits became a little less exact. And along with the Everyday Sadist strolled in other traits and types.

Soon, the Everyday Sadist became, simply, the Sadist. And the Dark Triad came to be known by other names, such as the Dark Core. And this Dark Core had even more traits—egoism, spitefulness, entitlement (all of which Paulhus and Jonason and other psychologists and researchers tried to keep separate from the original Dark Triad). The Dark Core then morphed into the "D-factor." A term that was coined by three European psychologists from Denmark's University of Copenhagen in their 2018 paper, "The Dark Core of Personality."

In a press release put out by the university, the paper and its authors declared that all these dark qualities of the Dark Tetrad, they're really just fueled by one thing: the D-factor. That's where all the traits emanate from, and it explains why the Psychopath shares some of his behaviors with the Narcissist, and why the Narcissist shares traits with the Machiavellian. They move in and out of each other, in a way. They're fluid. They interpret the D-factor as the unifying element, the thing where all these traits are stored, the element that allows these Dark types to do what they do without regard for anyone else but themselves. Almost an instinct, this factor serves as a kind of excuse for their behaviors.

On the psychologists' Dark Factor website, which features an attractive color wheel of all the various dark traits (Sadism, Psychological Entitlement, Moral Disengagement, etc.) in a rainbow of colors, in the center of which is a big white **D**, and which also offers a free questionnaire to determine your D-score, the three professors explain why they decided to rebrand Dark Psychology and the Dark Triad as the D-Factor:

What's useful and applicable about their definition of what exactly the D Factor is and how they want it to serve as the foundational glue of a unified theory of all these dark traits is their point about usefulness being at the root of what drives these individuals. Dark Personality types, selfishly, seem to believe that they have an inherent, biologically or almost spiritually driven need to express their darker desires and make those desires a reality. Even if it comes at the expense of others, they see their usefulness, in service to this D-factor, as superior to everyone else's. And at times, if their usefulness (pleasure) negatively affects the usefulness of someone else (i.e., others experience pain), they don't really care. Even worse, these folks who are giving expression to their D-factor, they are the opposite of altruists. They won't help a coworker cement a deal, they won't help a stranger change a tire, they can't even experience joy for someone else's achievements or happiness. Especially not if that other person's happiness can't in some way benefit them. Talk about selfish.

The D Factor is pretty much what most other researchers of Dark Psychology have been saying it is all along: the art (sometimes the science) of manipulation and mind control. It's people, people of different Dark Personalities (different Dark traits) employing motivation, persuasion, manipulation, and coercion to get what they want. Those tactics can also include brainwashing, mind control, lying and deception, concepts and actions that are sometimes standalone but often, like the Dark Personalities, almost indistinguishable from persuasion or coercion—or so overlapping with other characterological deficits and personality traits as to be almost inseparable. Almost all are liars, often pathologically so. And in terms of behavior, these Dark Personalities share many of the same traits—from consistent irresponsibility, cruelty, hostility, vanity, and impulsivity to a proneness for self-harm and addictions, interpersonal exploitation, emotional instability, perfectionism, anger, rage, and excessive defensiveness.

Similarly, most people trying to manipulate others are likely lying or trying to persuade them to do something (that they wouldn't otherwise want to do). Brainwashing is synonymous with mind control—it often just depends on how technical the methods are in employing one or the other. All of which can make it difficult to distinguish a Psychopath from a Machiavellian, an Everyday Sadist from a Narcissist, since, again, most Machiavellians and Psychopaths rely on deception and manipulation to achieve their ends, and many an Everyday

Sadist is also a Narcissist. Still, it's important, in terms of figuring out how to deal with these Dark Personalities, to determine who is what. While many people would assume that the convicted Ponzi schemer Bernie to be an unrepentant Psychopath, he's actually more of a corporate Machiavellian who relied on a deliberate, well-thought-out course of action for how to exploit others. Even an ingenious Psychopath—a true Psychopath, not just the subclinical variety—would need inordinate self-control to pull off the machinations Madoff did—especially over such a long period of time.

Admirable? Heinous? Forgivable? Unforgivable?

Some generalizations about the Dark Triad can, however, be made with a decent degree of certainty. For instance, many if not most celebrities are narcissistic (if not also, indeed, subclinical Narcissists). Most of the world's leaders are Machiavellian. And a decent amount of the most successful entrepreneurs, CEOs, business leaders, and entrepreneurs can safely be described as Psychopathic.

Uber's onetime CEO and founder Travis Kalanick, for instance, was described in *The Washington Post* as clinically sociopathic. As successful as Steve Jobs but worse in so many other ways, Kalanick seemed to have not only indulged his Shadow but given it steroids. Nasty steroids. And then let it loose, unchecked, on his coworkers, his competitors, his drivers, on reporters covering his industry, on whoever he seemed to feel got in his way. He was a Dark Personality nonpareil. And yet he thrived. People forgave him. They put up with his behavior. They indulged him and praised him.

Even so, what makes all this problematic is that there are just as many people confusing the issue of the Dark Triad by taking the position that these are not bad or negative traits but positive and even necessary. As *Entrepreneur* contributor Gene Marks stated about Kalanick, after acknowledging actions that included sexual harassment, threats to journalists, cutting Uber drivers' wages to below minimum wage, allegedly ordering and then cancelling thousands of fake rides for its competitor Lyft, and on and on—Marks still refused to see what the big deal was. The media, and his own shareholders and colleagues, many of whom were probably as guilty of all the things Kalanick was guilty of, or thought to be guilty of, or accused of having done, seemed to have turned on him just because of a few transgressions. Forgivable transgressions, Marks argued, in light of the fact that the guy had turned Uber into a global behemoth worth tens of billions of dollars. Why criticize him, Marks asked, why demand he resign and be put out to pasture, just for being who he is?

Which is sort of like excusing the alleged sexual assaults and otherwise execrable behavior of ex-Miramax co-founder and longtime Hollywood executive Harvey Weinstein because he'd produced so many Oscar-winners and blockbusters. Or giving a pass to R&B singer and music producer R. Kelly because he's the 55th best-selling music artist in the U.S., and collaborated with the likes of Jay-Z and Michael Jackson. Or trying to take any sort of sympathetic stance toward a convicted sexual predator—and Psychopath—like Larry Nassar, the former USA Gymnastics national team doctor who was sentenced to federal prison for 60 years and state prison for up to 145 years for the sexual assault of at least 250 girls and young women because of . . . what? He had a wife and children?

Women on the Verge

Not surprisingly, people tend to be more accepting of these Dark Triad/Tetrad traits in men as opposed to women. In the study, "Characters We Love To Hate: Perceptions of Dark Triad Characters in Media," which recently came out in the online issue of Psychology of Popular Media Culture, its authors showed participants film trailers of various movies to home in on how people perceive characters based on "Dark Triad" personality traits in relation to gender. Basically, they asked: Who do you prefer to watch?

Participants rated both Dark Triad and non-Dark Triad characters on likeability, relatability, appeal, and troublesomeness. Again not surprisingly, after analyzing the results, researchers found that:

—Non-Dark Triad female characters (the usual protagonists—low on narcissism, low on psychopathology) scored highest on likability, relatability and appeal, and scored lowest on the troublesome scale.

—Female Dark Triad characters rated lowest on appeal, likability and relatability and were seen as the most troublesome.

—Male non-Dark Triad characters came in higher in likeability and appeal and scored as slightly less troublesome than their Dark Triad counterparts.

In other words, Non-Dark Triad Men were: Tom Hanks—relatable but manly; Dark Triad Men: Clive Owen—more of a handful but still relatable; Non-Dark Triad Women: Jennifer Aniston—housewife-ish, girlfriend-y; Dark Triad Women: Angelina Jolie—trouble.

The authors concluded that the Dark Triad females were seen as more troublesome because these types aren't seen as often in the real world. Part of the reason being that the characteristics of the Dark Triad are usually ascribed to men, much less so to women, and so the Dark girls in the study went against what society considers to be . . . feminine.

The takeaway for Stephanie Ariganello, who wrote about this study for DearProducer.com, was as much about women inside the film industry as it was about the perception of cinematic female characters on the moviegoing public. It's OK for men of the Dark Triad to behave the way they have, and continue to do (despite the "successes" of the #MeToo movement), in Hollywood. It's OK for men to fight for their film ideas, their films, and have their stories told the way they want them told. But when women display this same tenacity and drive, they're labeled Narcissists. It's OK for men to engage in risky behavior, convincing other people to invest millions of dollars in their harebrained idea, and to follow through on that project with abnormally, off-puttingly laserlike focus. But when women do it, when they're overseeing something chancy, a big-budget movie that every other studio has passed on, they're called Psychopaths. And when men achieve all of this due to their gameplaying, their jaded outlook on everyone else in their industry, all the while lording their titled positions over everyone beneath them, they're given a pass. But when a woman does it, people whisper about what a Machiavellian bitch she is. Even though Machiaelli himself said that it was probably better to be feared than loved—women are pressured, it seems, into feeling like they have to be both.

Should women in the film industry, then, behave more like men? Are the ones in Hollywood not nice? Or assumed not to be nice? Are women in leadership in other industries expected to be just as womanly, just as unmanly as what Ariganello insinuates? Can women be like Jobs but still be likable? Studies show that men in business experience more praise than their female counterparts. Even men who would seem to be letting their Dark Traits peek out if not run the show. Even then, men tend to be seen as the kind of guy his employees and peers would want to hang out with. Maybe not regularly or often but they can relate to him.

Ariganello then brings out Marianne Cooper, who addressed the issues of likability and female leadership in the *Harvard Business Review*. What Cooper has found in many a study, over and over again, is the predictable double-standard for these women who've managed to make it in the business world. In particular, there's a backlash against those women who indulge their Dark Traits, who believe in that bumper sticker that says, Well-behaved women rarely make history. These are women who may be acting like men. But only certain kinds of men. Men a bit like Kalanick. Maybe not as egotistical and callous and self-serving as Kalanick, or even as monofocused and affectless as Jobs, but certainly modeling themselves, or maybe just giving into that D-factor deep down inside them.

Define Certifiable

Currently, only two of the three Dark Triad traits qualify as pathological: Narcissism and Psychopathy. The fourth one, the Everyday Sadist, which was added by Dark Triad co-originator Delroy Paulhus in 2014 to form the Dark Tetrad, continues to straddle the line of pathological and non-pathological. Pathological, in relation to psychology and Dark Psychology, and specifically as it relates to the Dark Triad (or Tetrad), means, according to the American Heritage dictionary, "relating to or caused by disease," or, "of, relating to, or manifesting behavior that is habitual, maladaptive, and compulsive."

To qualify as a pathological sadist, then, that person would have to exhibit behavior that typically caused by or related to a disease that leads to habits, adaptations, and compulsive issues. For a mental or psychological condition or behavior to be warranted as a disorder or disease, that usually means it's been granted such a status in the *Diagnostic and Statistical Manual of Mental Disorders*, the bible for all psychologists and psychiatrists published by the American Psychiatric Association. Now in its fifth edition, and known as the *DSM-5*, clinicians, researchers, drug companies and drug-regulation agencies, health insurance companies, the pharmaceutical industry, the legal system, and policy makers all rely on this tome to diagnose and treat clients and patients. To label someone insane or a Psychopath, on the one hand, while deciding not to include Sadism or Sadistic personality disorder in the *DSM* (it appeared as a personality disorder in the appendix of the *DSM-III*) is often subjective and controversial. (For example, the APA did not fully depathologize, and therefore normalize homosexuality until 1987. Until then, homosexuality had been listed in the *DSM* as a mental disorder.) As evidenced by the case of Uber's co-founder above: what's acceptable behavior and what's not? Who's certifiably Psychopathic and who's normal?

What's hard to argue against is that these Dark Personalities of the Dark Triad/Tetrad are traits that need to be treated, that are inherently undesirable (by and large socially condemned or personally counter-productive—despite the widespread support of characters like Kalanick by places like *Entrepreneur*). And when combined, these three (or four) traits can turn an otherwise tolerably annoying or problematic person into someone both dangerous and destructive, to themselves as well as others.

Chapter 3: The Machiavellian

Men are so simple of mind, and so much dominated by their immediate needs, that a deceitful man will always find plenty who are ready to be deceived.

Niccoló Machiavelli, *The Prince*

Named for Niccoló Machiavelli, author of the 16th century political treatise, *The Prince*, this trait is used to describe someone who's cunning, scheming and unscrupulous—and all the while showing almost no emotion, no feeling, no empathy for those who are being manipulated and deceived. Machiavellians are often detached—from themselves and from conventional morality, and fully believe that the ends justify the means—the means often being anything and everything.

In his book, Machiavelli provided a kind of blueprint on how to get to the top: strong rulers should be severe with their own people as well as their enemies, and glory and survival should be had no matter what the cost, and even if they were iniquitous and depraved.

Machiavellians often use coercion, persuasion, manipulation, deception, gaslighting, mind control, and mind games to achieve their goals—which are often all about attaining power or control. They tend to pursue money, power, and competition and agree with statements such as "Never tell anyone the real reason you did something unless it is useful to do so"—all while maintaining a "cool" or "cold" approach. They take a win-at-all-costs outlook on life, and frown on family commitment, self-love, and community building. They are charming but only facilely so, have no qualms about undermining others, show a high prevalence for depression, and can be sexually coercive and highly promiscuous.

Name any historical or current political leader and it's likely they're a Machiavellian—from Richard Nixon and Rudolph Giuliani to Vladimir Putin and Joseph Stalin, whose quotes are so perfectly Machiavellian they almost defy belief: "Death is the solution to all problems. No man—No problem," and "I trust no one, not even myself."

Shakespeare love Machiavellian characters (who appear throughout his historical plays), as do film and TV writers. Two of the more venal, most purely Machiavellian characters of the past two decades include Lord Baelish (aka Littlefinger) of *Game of Thrones*, who adheres to the Machiavellian philosophy that life is essentially a "ladder of chaos," and every opportunity to get ahead must be exploited, whether it's dispatching enemies, employees, co-conspirators, or kings, and Tony Soprano of *The Sopranos*, who maintains power at all costs, again, like Baelish, killing off rivals, co-conspirators, other bosses, or members of his own family, and who exemplifies Machiavelli's belief that "Since love and fear can hardly exist together, if we must choose between them, it is far safer to be feared than loved. Men are less careful how they offend him who makes himself loved than him who makes himself feared."

Also seen in those with Psychopathy and Narcissism, Machiavellianism is mostly about manipulating others for one's own gain. Other signs of Machiavellianism include:

- Frequent use of flattery
- A tendency to come off as aloof or hard to know
- A cynical attitude, especially when it comes to goodness and morality
- An inability to commitment and emotional attachments
- Because of their calculating nature, they can be extremely patient
- They rarely reveal their true intentions
- can be good at reading social situations and others
- They lack warmth and compassion
- They are not always aware of the consequences of their actions
- They can struggle to articulate their own emotions

- They have a knack for reading social situations and others

It's this last quality that can be most unsettling. As outlined in various studies that began to look at people with a high degree or highly developed level of emotional intelligence (high EQs), they discovered that EQ, being that it tends to be "morally neutral," can, taken to the extreme, turn out to be blatant Machiavellianism. A high EQ can be used for the protection and betterment of oneself and others, but it can also be exploited as a way to advance oneself ahead of others.

In a 2014 study led by University of Toronto psychologist Stéphane Côté, his team looked at university employees who'd scored high for both emotional intelligence and Machiavellianism. Côté then looked at how often these school workers shamed and belittled their fellow workers. The Machiavellians with the high EQs turned out to be the employees who partook in the most harmful behaviors.

In a previous study of EQ in relation to Machiavellianism, in a paper titled, "Strategic use of emotional intelligence in organizational settings: Exploring the dark side," Martin Kilduff, Chair of Organizational Behavior at University College London, wrote that high-EQ individuals exploit their EQ abilities to advance themselves in their company environment, over and above the costs to their fellow workers. More cynically, they seem to know they have higher EQ skills, and so they work them for all their worth. Like any good Narcissist, they hide their true feelings, pretend they're feeling something else—depending on what sort of emotion or emotions they see the situation calls for. In other words: they fake it. And because of their emotional intelligence, they're as cunning as a Iago or as Scar from The Lion King. They manufacture false emotions out of themselves to play with the emotions of others.

Perhaps the most notorious Machiavellian of late has been Bernie Madoff, the onetime non-executive chairman of the NASDAQ stock market, and admitted mastermind behind the largest Ponzi scheme in world history, and the largest financial fraud in U.S. history (a fraud estimated to have cost investors at least $64.8 billion). Despite possessing Psychopathic traits, Madoff does not qualify as an out-and-out Psychopath. A truly subclinical Psychopath would lack the self-control needed for pulling off schemes as long-term and sophisticated as those orchestrated by Madoff.

Hardly solace to anyone who was victimized by him, but as Paulhus has said of the Machiavellian: the Machiavellian, when he's fully engaged, is so good at what he does that the person or persons he's doing it to, they don't even realize it. In fact, they tend to praise the Machiavellian. Even as that Machiavellian character is slowly boiling them in water. Worse, the Machiavellian's capacity to manipulate tends to leave their victims doubtful of their own instincts, or feeling codependent and addicted to having them in your life.

Chapter 4: The Narcissist

The lion is most handsome when looking for food.

Rumi

"It is important to understand that most people have narcissistic pathology, so this is not to dismiss Jung. We all have narcissistic problems. Someone has suggested that we need a 'Humans Anonymous Twelve Step Program,' to help everyday people deal with their residual narcissistic pathology, and I agree. It's another way of saying that we need a more practical approach to our spirituality if we are to be effective in containing and channeling our grandiose energies."

Robert L. Moore, *Facing the Dragon: Confronting Personal and Spiritual Grandiosity*

Named after the character Narcissus in Greek mythology, the vain young man who fell in love with his own image reflected in a pool of water, in psychoanalytic terms, Narcissism came to fame via Sigmund Freud's 1914 essay "On Narcissism" and, since being classified as a personality disorder in the 1968 *DSM* (where it grew out of the concept of megalomania), this egotistic (though not egocentric) admiration of one's idealized self-image and attributes seems to be as appealing as it is vilified as a personality trait.

As a Dark Psychology trait it's the belief that you deserve and expect admiration and to be treated differently than others. Think Joan Crawford, Kanye West, Kim Kardashian, Mariah Carey, Madonna, Donald Trump, Jim Jones, Adolf Hitler. Narcissists all. Dark Narcissists. And as defined by Tomas Chamorro-Premuzic in an essay for the *Harvard Business Review* ("Why Bad Guys Win at Work"), Narcissism is huge in ways that wouldn't be so awful if they weren't so blown up to such unworldly proportions. Narcissists consider themselves better than everyone else—better at almost anything and everything, even at things that are way outside their wheelhouse. And they are so into themselves that no one else hardly exists. But they're also incredibly magnetic, entertaining, full of energy. Making them fun to be around, desired. People like having them around, despite how little they care about the welfare or health of anyone else. Jim Jones was a Narcissist. Italian media tycoon and former Prime Minister of Italy Silvio Berlusconi was a Narcissist. As was Jobs. History and the arts are full of Narcissists.

Sometimes referred to "normal narcissists," subclinical Narcissists usually exhibit a sense of entitlement and seek admiration, attention, prestige, and status. They also have a sense of perceived superiority to others and an intolerance to criticism, plus, they are high in dominance motivation—meaning, they demote and ostracize talented others, hoard information from the group (as a way to maintain their social rank), closely monitor others (to reduce any perceived threat to their social rank), prevent subordinates from bonding or teaming up with other group members, and often assign talented others to roles that are beneath their skill set (in order to prevent them from excelling).

Magical thinkers who see themselves as flawless, Narcissists tend to have no shame and very poor boundaries—their own or respect of others', as other people tend to be seen as just extensions of themselves, or they exist merely to serve the needs of the Narcissist (if they really exist at all). Being that there's hardly any border between self and other, it's not surprising that Narcissists, as well as Psychopaths and Machiavellians, tend to attract others—maybe not long-term but long enough to do damage, to pass on their genes to.

In a 2013 study that created high and low Dark Triad characters, and then obtained ratings from women scoring the attractiveness of these characters' personalities, characters with high Dark Triad personalities were found to be significantly more attractive to the women than ones with low Dark Triad personalities. The male character's Dark Traits were: self-interested, manipulative, and insensitive. A later study then found that women who were more strongly attracted to the faces of Narcissistic men tended to have more children. And in yet another study, which presented fictionalized versions of the opposite sex to participants, each character being a Narcissist, a Machiavellian, or a Psychopath, the Narcissists came off way better. Participants even thought some of them were "hot." The Psychopath and the Machiavellian? Not.

No wonder that Narcissists, who tend to have an unrestricted sociosexuality, find it easier to start new (and numerous) relationships, and have higher levels of infidelity. They tend to be commitment-phobic, with little interest or motivation to remain in existing or long-term relationships.

In an earlier, similar study, Mitja Back and Boris Egloff of Johannes Gutenberg-University of Mainz, along with Stefan Schmukle at Westfalische Wilhelms-University of Muenster, collected information on students' personalities and then had them briefly introduce themselves to one another. Students who'd scored higher on Narcissism were seen by others as more likable. The Narcissistic students were perceived as having flashier appearances, being more confident in their body language, and possessing more attractive facial expressions. Narcissists, it appeared, carried and presented themselves in ways that made for a better, more striking first impression.

Physical attractiveness, especially when combined with seemingly better social skills (more attentive, more polite, more solicitous), creates the so-called "halo effect," a kind of cognitive bias wherein we tell ourselves things such as "What is beautiful is good," or "He is nice!" ergo, "He is smart too!" Narcissists, who invest an inordinate amount of their energy into their looks and appearance, are doubly rewarded by this type of impression; and when humor and/or confidence are thrown in, two other qualities Narcissists pride themselves on, people are even more susceptible to forming a misleading impression.

And even though it's often only a matter of time until the Narcissist's game is found out, given that Narcissists and other Dark Personalities aren't usually built for long-term relationships, time can often be relative. Narcissists have plenty of tactics at their disposal to keep their victims in their thrall. And whoever falls for the Narcissist often continues to fall for other Narcissists.

In Martin Buber's words, the malignantly narcissistic insist upon "affirmation independent of all findings." Self-criticism is a call to personality change . . . The evil are pathologically attached to the status quo of their personalities, which in their narcissism they consciously regard as perfect. I think it is quite possible that the evil may perceive even a small degree of change in their beloved selves as representing total annihilation.

M. Scott Peck, *People of the Lie*

Narcissists: Unjust Players in a Just World

As people, over time (though not that long a time), they're also poor listeners, mean-spirited, "emotional cripples," and calculating. As partners, they're oppressive and crazy-making, leaving exes and former colleagues and friends and estranged family members feeling . . . crazy, most of all, but also hurt, confused, humiliated, subservient, degraded, demeaned, devalued, confused, lost, wrung out, sad, empty, fooled, played for a fool, abused, brainwashed, mistrustful, untrustworthy, suffocated, and sucked dry. As Paulhus casually if succinctly characterized them, they are the biggest P.T. Barnums—but for themselves—who can't ever get enough praise, enough screen time, enough adoration, enough ink. In the long run, they're boring. In the even longer run, people begin not to want them around at all, despite how entertaining they used to be.

But as stated above, Narcissists can also be extremely charming, funny, fun to be around, and seemingly normal. It's the normal part that, like the Machiavellian, the Psychopath, and the Everyday Sadist, they are geniuses at coming off as and exploiting in others. This is because they are especially good at picking up others' vulnerabilities and weaknesses— other people's sore spots. (Made all the easier if the Narcissist's mark is codependent.) Other people's shame. Their abusive backgrounds, their alcoholic parents, their Narcissistic brother, mother, uncle, sister. Their weight, their appearance, their finances. Their fear of being alone, their fear of not being loved.

Or if not their sore spots, they home in on whatever it is they love or value or fear losing the most: their children, their job, their hopes and dreams. These are all things that the Narcissist figures out in the early stages of a relationship—during what's called the "love bombing" and "good listener" phase.

And once they find out the things that are most important to a person, they zero in on those things, they use them against that person. Brutally. Mercilessly.

Dana Morningstar, a domestic violence educator who focuses on abuse awareness and prevention, and who's also been in a Narcissistic relationship, is one of the more insightful writers on the topic. She is also the author of *Out of the Fog: Moving from Confusion to Clarity After Narcissistic Abuse*, and has a blog, a podcast, and a YouTube channel (in addition to running several online support groups), all of which you can find under the name "Thrive After Abuse." In her online column, she writes about living with a Narcissist, and how it's fundamentally different from a normal relationship. Invoking the concept of the "Just World," a sociological notion that's kind of the Golden Rule—treat others the way you expect them to treat you. Only this Just World idea, Narcissists don't adhere to it. Not at all. (Or maybe a little, but only, only when it serves their selfish purposes.) Normal people, though, assume that most everyone else is normal. Evil people, they stick it. We know what they look like, how they treat other people. And Narcissists don't look at all evil. Or even bad. Why would this person not treat us the way we're treating them?

Therein lies the our mistake, and all the opportunity in the world for the Narcissist. In a relationship, the woman who chooses, unknowlingly, a Narcissist as her mate (if even only temporarily), when they run into something hurtful or unthinking from their mate, they dial in to their Just World playbook. Naturally, they think, they'll change. They'll be better. They know what they did was mean. That it brought me pain. But for Narcissists and Sociopaths, stresses Morningstar, who can't seem to stop bringing these Dark Personality types into her life, into her orbit, they just go mum. They do not change. They will not change. Change does not serve them. Especially when that particular behavior that harmed their partner, if that brought a weird kind of glee or excitement to the Narcissist, to the Sociopath, then leave or be prepared for more of it. Why? What does this infliction of pain to others, others they should seemingly care about or make an exception for (not be cruel to)? Because it's not only rewarding on the level of excitement, it worked so it must have value. It makes them feel important, superior. Better than. Which they already consider themselves better than everyone else, but the more they can prove this to themselves and, by extension, to others, the better the payout.

Many people who end up in a relationship with a Narcissist are people who grew up in a household with a Narcissist, or they have other issues they haven't fully worked out, such as self-esteem or self-worth—issues Narcissists feed on like so much chum. But others are just as susceptible to getting involved—and staying with—a Narcissist. People with no issues at all. People with decent self-esteem, and healthy self-worth. How? Why? Because they are normal. Because they trust others, they believe what other people tell them. Especially when those other people are seen holding the door open for an older woman, or stopping to help a stranded motorist fix their flat tire. All just part of the act. As Morningstar reflects about one of her past Narcissist boyfriends, he was kind. He was considerate. He was the type to help out little old ladies. He never criticized Morningstar. He seemed to share his feelings with her. He seemed to be transparent—of his actions, with his emotions. He never exposed her to the devaluing phase (the stage where you start wondering why someone who cares for you would possibly treat you as nastily as they do). He even enjoyed hanging out with kids and her friends. And he had a good sense of humor. Until. Until he didn't. Until he went narcissistically psycho on her.

Morningstar's point being that, even good, psychologically robust people, they too can fall for a Narcissist. And once these people have allowed a Narcissist into their life, the healthy person tends not only to stay, they overstay. Why? Because, as Morningstar puts it, people like her, people who know how to treat others, the way most people believe that it's a Just World, they don't even realize, they have an almost impossible time accepting that they are living with a Narcissist.

You will always be the prey or the plaything of the devils and fools in this world, if you expect to see them going about with horns or jangling their bells. And it should be borne in mind that, in their intercourse with others, people are like the moon: they show you only one of their sides. Every man has an innate talent for . . . making a mask out of his physiognomy, so that he can always look as if her really were what he pretends to be . . . and its effect is extremely deceptive. He dons his mask whenever his object is to flatter himself into some one's good opinion; and you may pay just as much attention to it as if it were made of wax or cardboard.

Arthur Schopenhauer,
Counsels and Maxims

When a Pipe Isn't a Pipe At All but a Really Big Red Flag

Like many people, Morningstar did not see the red flags her Narcissist had been waving—as red flags. She chalked up her Narcissist's behaviors as mistakes anyone could make (multiple kids outside of committed relationships, bankruptcy) or merely as signs of his lack of maturity (bounced checks, professing his love for her within two weeks of having met, an inability to plan ahead). And she took his explanations of all this, and his checkered past, at his word. So when she found out about his infidelity (with dozens of other people), his lies, his deceit, she was shocked.

She'd been raised, by society, based on her own cognitive bias, to look for other red flags—not the ones her Narcissist boyfriend had been letting loose. Fresh off a divorce, she'd been expecting issues around power and control, a bad temper, a guy who was a jerk to kids, a bad son, someone who treated waiters and bartenders dismissively, who kicked dogs. There was none of that. Naturally, she blamed herself. Where had she gone wrong? Why hadn't she seen this? Paid more attention to that? As she relates it, the only thing she could tell was that her ex was not like her, not like other decent folks. Especially his behavior. That was off-the-charts whack. At one point, she decided the man she'd brought into her life was a con artist.

What Morningstar also learned, about herself and about others like her, and most especially about Narcissists (and other Dark Personality types) was that we've been socialized to expect bad people to look and behave like they look and behave in the movies. Or in mug shots. Or the way they're so often portrayed on Lifetime. They aren't. Not in real life. They come off as great guys, maybe sometimes a little egocentric, a little juvenile. All of which Morningstar saw, in the tiniest of ways, early on. All of which she shouldn't paid more attention to. But she didn't. Damn that whole Just World thing. She shouldn't listened to her instincts. She should have been more skeptical. Not doubting. Just more careful. More concerned about her feelings, not the other person's. Because in a real relationship, a healthy one, each person can tell the other what they're feeling, what they like and don't like, what works and what doesn't work—and not be beaten up for expressing that. Not have the other person go into denial, or blame their partner. Or abuse them even more. In short, Morningstar learned to have healthier, stronger boundaries.

Malignant, Cerebral, Somatic

In another post from her Thrive After Abuse site, Morningstar defines three types of Narcissist: Malignant, Cerebral, and Somatic. Despite most victims' belief that a Narcissist is a Narcissist, researchers and clinicians and other professionals in the therapy world seem to think that not all Narcissists are the same. Further, more than a few argue that Narcissists exist on a spectrum (not unlike the spectrum for Asperger's/Autism). The Cerebral and Somatic Narcissists might be characterized as passive—or more passive than a Malignant Narcissist, who exhibits the classic traits of Narcissistic Personality Disorder, but in addition shows additional symptoms of Sadistic, Antisocial, and Paranoid Personality Disorders. Malignant Narcissists lack almost any empathy and rarely if ever show any remorse for whatever deliberately inflicted damage they've inflicted on others.

No matter, argues Morningstar. Narcissists can present just as much danger to a partner as the scariest of Psychopaths or Sociopaths. They're just as capable of snapping. They're quixotic. And they have no feelings for others, no sense of sorry if they do hurt others. Which means they have the potential to go from that of a passive-aggressive dweeb to full-on fatal in a heartbeat. Narcissists, no matter how seemingly nonthreatening they are, as Narcissists who rage on a regular basis.

While not as deliberately or overly aggressive or destructive, the Cerebral Narcissist and the Somatic Narcissist are centered, on sex and the body, respectively. The Cerebral Narcissist tends to use sex as a weapon. In the beginning of the relationship, they'll speed up the intimacy, but once they've got their partner in their clutches, they often cut off or suddenly slow down all sexual contact. This is part of what's known as Narcissistic supply: not the sex but the sexual partner. The Narcissist's partner, they are the Narcissistic supply. When that supply dries up, or leaves, even though it's the Narcissist who initiated the ending of all sexual intimacy, the Narcissist interprets that as a Narcissistic injury—a threat to their self-esteem or self-worth (and an injury that taps into their extreme sense of vulnerability). In return, the Narcissist can then lashes out in Narcissistic fury. The Cerebral Narcissist, though, tends to turn that fury inward. They'll gain weight, they'll quit caring about their physical appearance (often in order to further avoid any kind of intimacy). Instead of reaching out to their partner, they'll masturbate, or seek out prostitutes or one-night stands with strangers.

Somatic Narcissists are equally body-focused. Often found at the gym, or mulling over a visit to the plastic surgeon, or just obsessed with the latest fashions and what to wear, they base most of their energy and self-esteem on their appearance. Hypersexualized, they're often good at sex and wanting it often and from as many partners as will appreciate them. They can therefore often be found on dating websites and bars.

The persona is the mask we wear in relation to the world and others. It is created through a combination of socialization, societal expectations, one's experience of the world, and the natural attributes and tendencies of the individual. It combines elements of how we want to see ourselves, ideally, and how we want the world to see us, as well as how the world does see us and wants us to be. Our persona defines our social identity; it is constructed in relation to the roles we play in our lives and in our world, how we want to look and be seen. It is the face we wear to be presentable and acceptable to our society. It is not necessarily who we really are, but who we want and pretend to be to others and, many times, to ourselves.

David Schoen, *War of the Gods in Addiction*

Dr. Jekyll and Mr. Narcissist

Narcissists rarely change, but they do have many faces. Masks. Personas. Which can be misleading, not only in the beginning of a relationship with a Narcissist but at that point when their partner thinks they've changed. Narcissists rarely change their behavior for any prolonged length of time, and if it appears they have, it often means they've just gotten better at hiding things.

These faces that Narcissists show to the world—these are their public faces. The ones that are socially acceptable, nonthreatening, charming. And faces is too limiting. Narcissists have often perfected a role: the great parent, the volunteer, the churchgoer, world's best son, best spouse. Charming, witty, kind, considerate.

All pretense. All fake. All of which sounds bitter or cynical or beyond the pale of openmindedness and acceptance and forgiveness. Keep in mind, though, that these are Dark Personalities. Dark individuals with very Dark Traits.

When a Narcissist lets their guard down, when they give a glimpse behind the mask (behind the evil curtain), it's usually just their partner who sees it. And most often, it's not the Narcissist being vulnerable, being open with their partner—it's by accident. And the side of the Narcissist that's revealed, their

Dark Personality, it's often so unlike their public persona, so dark and ominous, the Narcissist's partner can hardly even comprehend what it is they're looking at, or being exposed to. Which, sticking to their Just World philosophy, they write off this darkness as a bad day. Despite it being an enormous red flag. Despite it being the Narcissist's true self: deceitful, manipulative, cold, callous, calculating, remorseless.

When, if ever, the Narcissist intentionally removes their public face, it's not till the so-called "discard" phase of the Narcissistic Abuse Cycle. As Morningstar puts it in no uncertain terms, once the Narcissist decides that your utility to them is done, you are essentially dead to them. So you may as well be dead. Which means, they're ready to find their next victim and probably don't care what level of damage they might do before they leave, so be extremely careful. By then, you are just in their way. You are no longer even a memory to them.

And given the prevalence and pervasiveness of domestic abuse, Morningstar is not being unreasonably melodramatic or inflammatory when she adds that no matter if a Narcissist has been mild-mannered his entire life. Once that veil slides away, once their true soulless personality has been revealed, once you are witness to that, to who they truly are, which, in truth, there's really no there there, there's really no emotive, compassionate human being inside them, they're just a shell, a husk, you better have an exit strategy in mind.

Emotional manipulation methodically wears down your self-worth and self-confidence, and damages your trust in your own perceptions. It can make you unwittingly compromise your personal values, which leads to a loss of self-respect and a warped self concept. With your defenses weakened or completely disarmed in this manner, you are left even more vulnerable to further manipulation.

Adelyn Birch, *30 Covert Emotional Manipulation Tactics: How Manipulators Take Control In Personal Relationships*

Aside from the Everyday Sadist, there is likely no better Dark Personality, or personality type or personality disorder, more masterful at manipulation. Particularly if and when they are covert about it.

Narcissists fit in. Even while seeming to stand out, they fit in with what the rest of society expects of its citizens: they are often successful at what they do (if not over the long haul), they are outgoing. They pretend to share the same values and morals as the rest of us—but only in order that that front allows them access to what they want: sex, attention, money, food, shelter, clothing, status.

The dark truth is they do not have the same morals and values as most other people. The non-Narcissists. They actually have no morals, no values whatsoever. They know what they are, sure, but they have no emotional or psychological connection to them. And often, to hide their deep abyss of immorality, they will go to great lengths to prove to the world that they have even higher moral standards, more solid values than anyone else. How? They're a deacon at their church. They volunteer at the local shelter. They lash out at people who demonstrate the least egregious amount of moral or ethical impropriety. They feed off the goodwill of others.

In short, they're emotional vampires. Sentient flimflammers. All the things they're railing against are the exact things they're most guilty of—think Bill Cosby, Jim Bakker, Scott Peterson. These men got away with all the things they did, despite the heinousness of their crimes. Because the rest of us, the women these men victimized, weren't just taken in by their celebrityhood, but assumed them to be good men, decent, normal men who would never take advantage of another human being in the ways that they did. This is why it takes so long for people to call them out for who and what they really are: we don't allow men like these into our lives, so to say that these men exist in our world, that makes no sense. And they prey on exactly that outlook that so many others have.

Even when we do snap out of it, most of us feel, again, that these men, these Narcissists, they can get better. And we can help them get better. They're too smart, too talented, too kind, too normal not to be as kind and loving and fun to be around as they were when they first swept us off our feet. This fix-it tendency can go on for months, sometimes years. Some people never do leave. But that doesn't mean the Narcissist got better, or changed his ways.

When a normal relationship keeps coming up against the same issues over and over, and those issues are never addressed or resolved, in time, it's clearly not a normal relationship. It's something else. That something else is usually one person not wanting to change, and the other person being manipulated.

When that's the case, it's not a normal relationship at all, it's an emotionally abusive relationship.

What Narcissist Really Really Love—Aside from Themselves

And this is the Narcissist's wheelhouse. This is where they thrive, what they live for, what they feed off of. (As long as the supply is still there, as long as they can keep the mask on.) Narcissists, being the master manipulators that they are—they know precisely what they are doing. They totally have the ability to control themselves. But do they want to? No. Never. As Morningstar says, again speaking from too much personal experience:

They *love* being this way. They thrive off of the thrill of keeping you sucked in, and they thrive off the thrill of following their every whim. (This is why their behavior is "erratic" and doesn't make any sense to anyone but them!) *But a person can only manipulate you if you let them. The easiest way to not be manipulated is to see their manipulation techniques for what they are.* Once you realize what they are doing isn't sincere, and is instead a series of calculated moves, you'll be less inclined to fall for them.

Which is why Morningstar set down what she sees as a Narcissist's favorite manipulation techniques, included below.

Denial. When confronted with their bad behavior, a Narcissist will generally deny that it ever happened—even if you confront them with hard evidence! If you can get them to admit to anything, they will generally only admit to the bare minimum, and deny that what they did was that bad, or to the extent that you think it really did happen. Victims stay sucked in because the manipulative person won't own their behavior— then the victim begins to question their own perceptions of what they saw. Because Narcissists and Sociopaths are such master manipulators, and are well-known for using a multitude of "gaslighting" techniques, that the victim is often more inclined to believe them rather than their own eyes.

Triangulation. Triangulation can happen in any dynamic that involves three people: at work, with children, with friends, you name it. A triangle is created with two other people that the Narcissist pits against each other to where the other people believe that each other are the problem, and not the Narcissist. This can be done with a Narcissistic parent pitting two of their children against each other, or with a Narcissist pitting his wife and the other woman against each other. This is a great trick, and works to keep the blame off of the Narcissist, as well as creates an ego feeding frenzy for them. They get their kicks from other being fought over (wife vs. the other woman), or from knowing that they have enough power and control to upset people to such an extent that they cause a lot of conflict and stress.

Pity. A Narcissist knows that if they can get you to feel sorry for them, then they can manipulate you into switching your focus from their bad behavior to all their trauma or other underlying reasons for their behavior. They'll try to get you to focus on their bad childhood, stress at work, their alcoholism, maybe their terrible ex-wife, or how depressed they've been. They may tell the victim that they are suicidal, need to go to rehab or detox, or perhaps that they think they have cancer. There are no lengths that these manipulators won't go to, and many times their pity inducing stories aren't even real.

Guilt. It's all your fault. Somehow in some way, his cheating, lying, and other bad behavior is also your fault. Perhaps he's telling you that you needed to be home more, or to spend more time with him, lose weight, gain weight, dress sexier, dress less sexy—whatever. According to him, his behavior is your fault. (This is the classic, "Look at what you made me do" cry of an abusive or manipulative person.) Because there is often a nugget of truth in every lie a Narcissist tells, the partner might fall for the guilt trip, and try to make sure they do better next time.

Intimidation. Intimidating behavior doesn't have to always be physical. It can be in the form of threatening to tell the courts that you are an unfit parent, and that they are going to go for full custody, or that if you divorce them that they'll go after your retirement. Of course, they might also stalk, or otherwise physically intimidate you as well–by hurting you, or by hurting objects around you (punching holes in walls, or breaking things), to scare you enough into letting them return to your life. Victims often stay because they are too scared to go, and they often feel like they are safer staying so they can at least know what the Narcissist is up to.

Hope. Narcissists do such an Oscar-winning performance of getting their victims to believe that this time they really will change, that it's understandable as to why the victim keeps believing them.

Morningstar then returns to the Just World philosophy. Normal people in normal relationships rightfully thinking that in a Just World, in a normal relationship when one person does something hurtful to the other, that person is sorry for their actions. In a Narcisstic relationship, when the non-Narcissist has been hurt, or experienced multiple issues of bad behavior, they continue to apply their Just World approach: This time they'll be different. They'll see how badly they've behave, how much damage they've caused. They'll change. They have to. This last episode was just too much, too awful.

There's no way they could possible do anything worse. That was rock bottom. They can't go any lower than that. They couldn't possibly be any meaner, any less compassionate. And therein lies the ultimate Narcissist trap: they can always up their game. They can always go lower. By then, the victim has put up with so much, there's almost no chance she'll ever have enough self-esteem or self-worth or self-confidence to leave. And so it worsens. Even when it felt like it'd never get worse.

So is there ever any hope for a relationship with a Narcissist? Morningstar is unequivocal: Not a chance. Narcissists will never modify their behavior. The only out is for the victim to change their behavior. And that's because the Narcissist sees nothing wrong with how they treat people. Even people they supposedly love. This speaks to the limitless sense of entitlement. It speaks to the fact that for the Narcissist, this is how they've always treated people, it's always worked (until it doesn't), and by the way, you chose to be with me.

Escaping the clutches of a Narcissist isn't easy. They will tell you everything you want (and need) to hear in order to keep you as their supply. They will appeal to both your pity and your hope that they will change given enough therapy, rehab, chances, or time at church. If this approach doesn't work, they will turn their issues back on you. They will manipulate you into feeling crazy, questioning if perhaps you are the one with the problem—that maybe you do have issues with trust, or with men, or with commitment or attachment. Or they may even flat-out deny that there is any issue to begin with. . . . The only thing worse than all the damage they've done, all the crap they've put people through, is their utter inability to feel or express the slightest amount of regret or compassion.

Chapter 5: The Psychopath

Not all psychopaths are in prison—some are in the board room.

> Robert Hare, "The Predators Among Us"

Although technically not a disorder, the Psychopath, someone characterized by persistent antisocial behavior, a lack or absence of empathy and/or remorse, egotistical, lacking in self-restraint, can be found in the *Diagnostic and Statistical Manual of Mental Disorders* under the diagnosis of Antisocial Personality Disorder (or as Dissocial Personality Disorder, which tends to be the official term for those types otherwise known as Sociopaths).

Subclinical psychopaths, as defined by Peter Jonason, author of the aforementioned Dark Triad study and the resident expert in Individual Differences and Evolutionary Psychology at Australia's University of Western Sydney, are characterised by high impulsivity and thrill-seeking and tend to have low empathy. Some (in)famous Psychopaths would include Tom

Cruise and Mel Gibson, Woody Allen and Donald Trump; toward the darkest end of the scale these would be the worse of the worst: Ted Bundy, Ed Gein (inspiration for the psycho killer in *Psycho*), Charles Manson, BTK serial killer Dennis Rader, and Jeffrey Dahmer.

These are the most heinous of Psychopaths, of course, and there are many other examples from throughout history (Heinrich Himmler, Adolf Eichmann, Josef Mengele, Ivan the Terrible, Vlad the Impaler, et al), but not all Psychopaths are violent. As Dark Triad enthusiast Delroy Paulhus has pointed out in his "Taxonomy of Dark Personalities" paper, they are easily the meanest, but that doesn't mean they're always out to physically hurt people. In his table of key features of the Dark Tetrad, Psychopaths score high on callousness, impulsivity, manipulativeness, and grandiosity. But unlike the Machiavellian, who lacks any outstanding quality of impulsiveness, Psychopaths are rarely involved in white-collar crimes. When others get in their way, they can become violent; although, again, not all Psychopaths turn to physical violence. But as Paulhus notes, there are many people whose Psychopathy remains low enough to keep them out of jail, though high enough to damage those they bring into their orbit.

Or, as stressed by Kevin Dutton, research psychologist at Magdalen College, University of Oxford and author of *The*

Wisdom of Psychopaths: What Saints, Spies, and Serial Killers Can Teach Us about Success, just because you're a Psychopath doesn't mean you're going to end up in jail.

Bigger, Stronger—More Evil, More Defined

In his groundbreaking 1941 book, *The Mask of Sanity*, Psychopathy champion and pioneer Hervey Cleckley (who would later overshadow his own work in the field of Psychopathy with his case study of a female patient, published as a book in 1956 and turned into the movie, *The Three Faces of Eve*, in 1957—which popularized another controversial mental diagnosis, that of Multiple Personality Disorder) declared Psychopaths as seemingly normal folks who can be engaging but whose "mask," like that of the Narcissist, hides a disturbingly ugly mental disorder.

In that same book, Cleckley also points out that this "normality" was especially present in the Psychopathic businessman who works industriously and subsumes his personality to that of the organized system—except when he's not, when he indulges his Psychopathy with periodic escapes into cheating on his wife, getting drunk, challenging others to a fight. As a prelude of sorts to the impending corporatism of the Company Man, and the stultifying and sometimes unpleasant compromises many men found themselves giving into in order to succeed in the expanding American business world, Cleckley foresaw the most dangerous consequences of how this life as a Yes man would play out in our culture over the coming decades.

As pervasive as Psychopaths soon became culturally and societally (from the popularity of Alfred Hitchcock's *Psycho*, released in 1960, to Charles Whitman, the "Texas Tower Sniper" who in 1966 killed 16 people in one afternoon to the 1971 conviction of cult leader Charles Manson to the rise of serial killings in the 1980s), it would still take another 40 years, and the work of another ambitious criminal psychology researcher, the University of British Columbia professor Robert Hare, before Psychopathy would cement its standing in the mental disorder industry. In 1981, Hare, frustrated by there not being an agreed-upon definition or rating system for Psychopathy, developed his own scoresheet. Known as the Hare Psychopathy Checklist, which drew heavily from Cleckley's list of Psychopathic traits, this assessment tool soon became the gold standard for measuring Psychopathy. In 1985, Hare upgraded the test and renamed it the Hare Psychopathy Checklist—Revised (known in criminology circles as the PCL-R). In Hare's diagnostic, which consists of all of 20 questions, the entry-level score for your garden-variety Psychopath is 27, with 40 being the highest possible. Most normal people come in at 2.

As used and interpreted by clinical psychologists, the PCL-R can be broken down into a four-factor model. These four dimensions are:

Interpersonal Items: Glibness and superficial charm; grandiose sense of self-worth; pathological lying; and conning/manipulativeness

Affective Items: Lack of remorse or guilt; shallow affect; callous/lack of empathy; failure to accept responsibility for their own actions

Lifestyle Items: Need for stimulation/proneness to boredom; parasitic lifestyle; lack of realistic, long-term goals; impulsivity; irresponsibility

Antisocial Items: Poor behavioral controls; early behavioral problems; juvenile delinquency; revocation of conditional release; criminal versatility

Corporate Psychos

The combination of low risk aversion and lack of guilt or remorse, the two central pillars of psychopathy may lead, depending on circumstances, to a successful career in either crime or business. Sometimes both.

By this time, as Wall Street went through an unprecedented boom in the 1980s, and its players came to be known and emulated as Masters of the Universe, despite epitomizing the me-first attitude sweeping through the corporate world and elsewhere, despite the sense of isolation and alienation that lurked beneath the false security of our consumerist culture, despite all of this being held up for question in books like *American Psycho* and movies like *Wall Street*, in the world of criminology and Psychopathic research, the white collar workplace became an arena of intense study. And out of these studies came the revelation that the corporate world was where the Psychopath felt most at home, where he (Psychopaths are predominantly male) not only felt comfortable but flourished. And was rewarded for his behaviors and predilections.

When Hare teamed up with industrial psychologist Paul Babiak, the result of their research was *Snakes in Suits: When Psychopaths Go to Work* (2006). In *Snakes*, Hare and Babiak described a five-phase model of how a typical workplace Psychopath rises to the upper levels and stays there. In the manipulative phase (Phase 3), the Psychopath creates for himself a working façade, one that'll fool those around him while not taxing him too much or totally inhibiting his

Psychopathic tendencies—what he, and a number of researchers, consider to be his good points. This fiction might involve the construction of themselves (to their coworkers and management) as trustworthy and sincere before moving in for the con. This fiction also involves the spreading of disinformation about potential rivals and critics and the setting up of the Psychopath as the nexus in a world of pawns and patrons (potential targets), who are then groomed into accepting the Psychopath's agenda.

As Hare told Dutton in *The Wisdom of Psychopaths*, there are undoubtedly a lot of Psychopathic players in the corporate world. More so, proportionately, than are found elsewhere. That's because Psychopaths gravitate to environments where they're not only able to exercise power and control over others, but they can strut their stuff statuswise as well, and even better, find lucrative financial reward too. Babiak, Hare's *Snakes in Suits* co-author, agreed. Because Psychopaths adapt so quickly to chaos and environments that are shifting so fast and so unpredictably, this is their wheelhouse. Their bliss, so to speak. They have access to all the stimulation they could ever desire, and even better, they can treat people as poorly and inconsiderately as they want, and people don't bat an eye. People even seem to respect them all the more. They're in Psychopathic heaven.

Even the language suits the Psychopath's purposes. A language most Psychopaths speak fluently and across cultures. Corporatese, workplace jargon, commercialese, corporate speak—the patois of boardrooms and bureaucracies—perfectly expressed the underhanded communications methods of the upwardly mobile Psychopath: a lack of clarity, tedious, difficult to understand, and opaque in its intentions.

Around that same boom time, however (the boom in Psychopaths, on Wall Street, in the cultural and criminological fascination with Psychopaths), Emory University psychology professor Scott Lilienfeld and his colleague and collaborator Brian Andrews, had become disenchanted with and frustrated by the PCL-R's lack of specificity. Lilienfeld and his colleagues saw Psychopathy the way scientists and other medical professionals had begun to see Asperger's and Autism: it's on a spectrum. Which is why some people will have some of the Dark Traits, but not all. Which was what led to the the genesis of the Psychopathic Personality Inventory (PPI), which consists of 187 questions.

Originally designed in 1996 as a self-report scale (as opposed to an interview-based assessment) for assessing the Psychopathic traits in non-criminal populations (usually among university students), but also of use in clinical populations (prisons and other institutions), and later revised in 2005 (and known as the PPI-R), there are eight distinct personality dimensions, or states, come together, which divide and reform along three superordinate axes. The states are: Machiavellian Egocentricity, Impulsive Nonconformity, Blame Externalization, Carefree Nonplanfulness, Fearlessness, Social Potency, Stress Immunity, and Coldheartedness; and the axes are: Self-Centered Impulsivity, Fearless Dominance, and Coldheartedness.

James Bond: Psychopath

Sentiment is a chemical aberration found on the losing side.

Sherlock Holmes

Given that an estimated 1 to 2 percent of the population qualifies as Psychopathic, researchers saw a potential breeding ground, or home, for Psychopaths in the business world; and estimates of Psychopaths in the corporate and business world were said to be as high as 3 percent. If there were so many Psychopaths in business, and overseeing the top tiers of businesses and corporations, then Psychopathy can't be all that bad. When Hare gave the PCL-R to 200 top U.S. business executives in 2010, the execs came out ahead and Psychopathy was positively associated with in-house ratings of charisma and presentation style: creativity, good strategic thinking, and excellent communication skills. And British psychologists Belinda Board and Katarina Fritzon, in 2005, found a greater preponderance of psychopathic traits among a sample of CEOs than they did among the inmates of a secure forensic unit.

In these years, the general tenor of studies tended to favor Psychopaths and their assorted traits. In 2010 Hideki Ohira, a psychologist at Nagoya University and his doctoral student Takahiro Osumi, discovered, in their glowingly titled paper, "The Positive Side of Psychopathy: Emotional Detachment in Psychopathy and Rational Decision-making in the Utimatum Game," that, when the decision-making of college students were examined while playing the ultimatum game, which illustrates the conflict between fairness and economic utility, psychopaths made better financial decisions than non-Psychopaths. Unfair offers did not bother them, nor did inequity. In the end, their indifference to the effects of the deal being painful or bruising to their ego did not matter; they ended up richer than the non-Psychopaths.

In that same year, New Mexico State University pychologist Peter Jonason reappeared as co-author of another pro-Psychopath paper, "Who Is James Bond? The Dark Triad as an Agentic Social Style." Basing their thesis on the attributes of Ian Fleming's international spy, they argued that men with a specific triangulation of Dark Personality traits—the Narcissist's unrepentant self-esteem; the Psychopath's thrill-seeking mercilessness; and the Machiavellian's guile and dishonesty—actually fare rather well in certain societal settings. Even more appealing to budding Psychopaths, these James Bonds were likelier to have more sexual partners and a stronger chance of hooking up randomly and often. Why? Psychopaths tend to lack the neuroticism and anxiety that impedes the undashing Joe Schmoes of the world from getting the girl.

It's studies like these that further mythologize the admiration for Psychopathic CEOs and lawyers, or, as it turns out, those who are carriers of the so-called "warrior gene" (also referred to in some circles as the "criminal gene"), monoamine oxidase A polymorphism (MAOA-L). Up until the mid-2000s, a deficiency in the *MAOA* gene was thought to lead to higher levels of aggression in males. Rebranded the "warrior gene" at one point, because a variant of it seems to be responsible for impulsive and aggressive behavior, there are those who have reframed it in an even more positive light, claiming that it causes its carriers to be more willing to take risks while simultaneously enabling them to better assess their chances of success in critical situations.

Psychopaths, it turns out, can seemingly teach us how to be better at certain things, in certain situations. Some of them, like autistics, are high-functioning. They can move through the world and be of use in it without being as damaging as their more malevolent brethren. And some have just learned to contain their darker emotions, their meaner ways.

Psychopath x Non-Psychopath = Success?

But then the pendulum swung again the other way.

In that same year as the other, more glowing reports on Psychopaths, Australian Clive Boddy, professor of management at the University of Tasmania and author of *Corporate Psychopaths: Organizational Destroyers*, served as the lead author on a study that wanted to know if employees viewed the corporate Psychopaths in their workplace midst as being good for Corporate Social Responsibility (CSR), or bad for it. After focusing on 346 corporate employees in Australia in 2008, Boddy and team found that the corporate Psychopaths were not only bad for business but bad for morale, bad for the workplace, bad for the community, and worse, the employees felt under-recognized, undervalued, underappreciated, and not remunerated in ways that reflected what they saw as their value to the company.

Undoubtedly, true Psychopaths, even subclinical Psychopaths of Dark Psychology, more often make for not-so-great leaders. Just as undeniable, though, is that Psychopaths do provide non-Psychopaths with traits that can be worth emulating. Though, like everything, in moderation. As Dutton wisely puts it in *The Wisdom of Psychopaths*, if a Psychopath increases his Psychopathy volume knob, letting it all out is as bad (for him and everyone around him) as it is to keep that Psychopathy entirely in check. When the Psychopath can keep himself at an even keel, between full-no Psychopathy and no Psychopathic behaviors at all, he's a healthy contributor to society. He's an alright guy. He's acceptable, even. OK to have around. And according to Dutton, the non-criminal Psychopath would, in an equation that might be worth considering, look like this:

Functional psychopath = (psychopath – poor decision making)

Context

More convincing than this somewhat practical-advice equation is when Dutton points out the overlaps between Psychopathic traits and spiritual traits: Non-attachment, focus and altered state of consciousness, energy, stoicism—all qualities shared by Psychopaths and Buddhism. He also lays out a program of his own, his Seven Deadly Wins—a kind of program that incorporates, in very modified terms, and with a lot of monitoring and self-monitoring, the essential qualities that make for a rather decent, beneficial version of a Psychopath. These Seven Wins can help the rest of us non-Psychopaths do better as individuals, teach us how to better handle Psychopaths, and do so in a way that's not at all Psychopathic or off-putting.

Dutton's Seven Deadly Wins are:

Ruthlessness

Charm

Focus

Mental toughness

Fearlessness

Mindfulness

Action

Most recently, Christian Jarrett, editor of the Research Digest blog published by the British Psychological Society, published a roundup piece on *Aeon* in which he made the rather bold if not entirely substantiated declaration that people prefer, even elect leaders who have the Dark Traits of the Psychopathic. As justification for this statement, he relied on a recent study from American personality psychologist Dan McAdams, in which Adams looked at the appeal of Donald Trump in an effort to understand his appeal. Trump's success, it seems, has to do with his overt aggression, his unceasing insults, the threats, the bullying. People respond to it. In part not just because some people aspire to be that rude and not be held accountable for it, but because our culture has been rewarding these types of Dark Personality types for decades now. It works. So why wouldn't we extol it?

Jarrett seems to feel that McAdams's take on Trump is part of a larger pattern. There's been a shift in who we admire and emulate. In short, voters tend to elect ineffective leaders with Psychopathic traits, which, as Jarrett interprets it, means that Psychopathy generally correlates with poorer leadership.

Boddy, the Australian author of *Corporate Psychopaths*, sure thinks so. But he's way down on this unchecked swing of the pendulum. Psychopaths are bad for business, period. In companies run by Psychopaths, or where Psychopaths are given free reign, the best employees, the most talented, tend to doubt their abilities, their ideas. They're shouted down. They're demeaned. They leave. They move on to businesses where there are no Psychopaths running the proverbial asylum. Businesses suffer. People suffer.

As proof of how individuals seem to gravitate toward those professions that are most suited for their Psychopathic or Non-Psychopathic Personalities, the results of the Great Britain

Psychopath Survey, based on people who'd completed the Levenson Self-Report Psychopathy Scale, were telling. On the left are the most Psychopathic professions, and on the right the least:

Most Psychopathic	**Least Psychopathic**
CEO	Care aide
Lawyer	Nurse
Media (TV/Radio)	Therapist
Salesperson	Craftsperson
Surgeon	
Beautician/Stylist	
Journalist	Charity Worker
Police Officer	Teacher
Clergyperson	Creative Artist
Chef	Doctor
Civil Servant	Accountant

Business or Pleasure?

Language and words for psychopaths are only word deep; there is no emotional colouring behind it. A psychopath can use a word like, 'I love you' but it means nothing more to him than if he said, 'I'll have a cup of coffee.'

Robert D. Hare, developer of
the Hare Psychopathy Checklist

Moving from the boardroom to the bedroom, Psychopaths behave even worse. If Psychopaths seem to move through the corporate world without a conscience, which many people excuse with the justification that it's not personal, it's business, the Psychopath is no more conscientious when it comes to romance or personal relationship. In fact, they're pretty much like the White Walkers of *Game of Thrones*: ice cold, no empathetic feelings, no connection.

Ironically, Psychopaths have no trouble seducing potential partners—after all, that's what they excel at: the pursuit, conquest, triumph. And it's not that Psychopaths avoid sex or aren't good at it, it's that it's largely performative. Forever goal-oriented, the sex, like the romance, is only worth having if the Psychopath has a worthy enough goal. Not particularly promiscuous though hardly chaste, but not at all into something long-term, for the Psychopath, sex and relationships are, according to Los Angeles clinical psychologist Seth Myers, what Psychopaths turn to not for a dopamine release but to jack up their ego. Or they're about power. Control. Or somehow more depressingly, it's what they resort to when they're overwhelmed with a kind of existential boredom.

This is why Psychopaths love to troll bars and restaurants, especially during happy hour. This is when a Psychopath's prey are more susceptible to excessive flattery, extremely personal questions, professions of an extremely deep, extremely destined connection—all happening incredibly fast. And because Psychopaths are especially gifted at recognizing emotions in others, as well as having an enhanced ability for faking their own emotions, those who are vulnerable (just out of a previous relationship, reeling from the death of a loved one, loss of a job) are even more vulnerable. Psychopaths, rather than having an impairment in recognizing the emotions of others, indeed have a talent for it.

Relationships of Inevitable Harm

Women often feel ridiculous that they let someone this disordered into their lives and they didn't even recognize the symptoms until she was way in over her head and emotionally destroyed. Welcome to the world of psychopathy where many—even most—don't recognize them either! The main characteristic of this disorder is social behavior and social hiding. Psychopaths blend in as 'normal' and manipulate others into believing them. These chameleon-like traits help them to move about freely and remain largely undetected.

> Sandra L. Brown, *Women Who Love Psychopaths: Inside the Relationships of Inevitable Harm With Psychopaths*

As articulate as Dana Morningstar when it comes to relationships with Narcissists, Sandra L. Brown is equally articulate and insightful when it comes to Psychopaths and their relationships, and especially when it comes to women in pathological relationships. Author of *Women Who Love Psychopaths: Inside the Relationships of Inevitable Harm*

With *Psychopaths, Sociopaths & Narcissists* and *How To Spot a Dangerous Man Before You Get Involved,* and founder of The Institute for Relational Harm Reduction & Public Pathology Education, Brown is not only wise to the evil ways of the Psychopath, she has a theory, the best and most cogent and convincing theory out there, about why Psychopaths continue to attract partners. (And though she logically speaks of Psychopaths as men, since male Psychopaths outnumber female Psychopaths almost four to one, her theory is just as applicable to male Psychopaths stalking male partners, or female Psychopaths stalking female partners.)

Describing the feeling of having succumbed to a Psychopath as the kind of experience not unlike having been mugged, throughout her work and her writing, Brown focuses almost exclusively on the victims and survivors. Not only because those are the people she most wants to help (as she says, again and again, Psychopaths are all but irredeemable), but because their stories rarely get told, and because through these women we get a much clearer picture of how Psychopaths worked their evil magic, what their tactics actually were, what type of women they prey on. As she put it in one of her online blogs: There's no chance of changing something that we can't diagnose. There's no way to deal with it effectively. And until we really figure out this whole Dark Psychology thing, until we have a working idea of what makes a Psychopath tick, we won't be able to help anyone else.

Women, she says, misjudge the Psychopath's pathology because of his prolific brain-games. He'd used gaslighting techniques to convince her she had a break with reality. He employed coercion and psychological warfare techniques. Some survivors called it 'The Ultimate Mind Screw'—sending prominent female executives, attorneys, and doctors into mental institutions to recover from him. Many showed signs of Stockholm Syndrome (the condition that causes hostages to develop a psychological alliance with their captors as a survival strategy during captivity), and most of the survivors she interviewed and treated felt like they'd been cut up by a chainsaw-wielding mindfucking follower of ISIS—only with a smile on his face and roses at the ready.

In her book, *Women Who Love Psychopaths*, she covers the Psychopath's tastes, his methodology, his techniques, and the wreckage he leaves in his wake. Cleverly stalking and wooing his prey, the Psychopath often stays just out of reach of law enforcement. Once ensnared, the victim feels caught, cruelly, in a device of her own making: self-preservation. And still there's the dichotomy between the pull of his charisma versus her loathing of him, the intense attraction, even trance and suggestibility.

In *How to Spot a Dangerous Man Before You Get Involved*, Brown focused on wreckage caused by these Dark Personality types, consequences characterized by dramatic, overly emotional or unpredictable thinking or behavior and interactions with others, disorders such as antisocial personality disorder, borderline personality disorder, histrionic personality disorder and narcissistic personality disorder, and what these do to a relationship. Here are some of the things she discovered:

- Educated and otherwise well-adjusted women described entrancement or 'vortexing' into relationships with psychopaths who have extraordinary skills for exploiting the suggestibility of others. [Most disturbingly, the victim is drawn, over and over again into the "vortex" of his power play.]
- The psychopath lured them through a form of hypnotic induction into trance states which contributed to how strongly women can be 'held' in these relationships.
- The role of intensity of attachment and fear affected her perception of sexual and relational bonding with psychopaths.
- The 'Jekyll and Hyde' dichotomous personality of the psychopath coupled with 'crazy-making' relationship dynamics aided the development of cognitive dissonance in the victims, weakening an otherwise strong emotional constitution.

- The victim aftermath symptoms either resembled or were in fact post-traumatic stress disorder (PTSD), even without physical violence.

As enlightening as this all is, though, what's truly helpful is the revelation Brown shares about how and why women are so susceptible to Psychopaths. Especially smart women. Accomplished women. Autonomous women with plenty of friends—male and female. Women with high self-esteem, secure jobs, self-confidence, strong, open relationships with their parents, and backgrounds one would never think would set them up as the future victim of a Psychopath. Brown's insight is this: the "Super Traits."

The Psychopath's victims possess a litany of traits that dovetail with the Psychopath's. As Brown sees it, the more autonomous the woman, the bigger the challenge to the Psychopath. The bigger the trophy she is as a conquest. He really has to be not just good but great, one of the greatest, if he's going to fool this woman, this woman who's achieved so much, who has no issues, no lack. And, perhaps, plenty of fringe benefits to go after: money, sex, material possessions. Friends who might be as well-off and as much of a challenge as well.

It's brilliant. It's cruel. It's cruelly ironic. Essentially, it's unjust and unfair. Yet it happens. And this insight of Brown's should be getting far more play than what little it has. In listening to these women's tales of Psychopathic possession, Brown understands that these Super Traits of theirs represents the kind of conquest to a Psychopath that's practically irresistible. Although the quote below would appear to be more applicable to that of the Everyday Sadist, it's really more appropriate here because of how soul-crushing it is.

Our sense of power is more vivid when we break a man's spirit than when we win his heart.

Eric Hoffer, *The Passionate State of Mind*

The Psychopath doesn't just seek out any partner, any woman. Not as his most self-celebratory conquests. As often as he may bed down indiscriminately, what he's really after is something memorable. A woman who offers not just a challenge but who, after having been subjugated, exists in his mind much the same way a serial killer relishes his trophies—souvenirs of his victims that he keeps, either physically or as a memory. And these unique women, whatever their Super Traits are, they're like the socket to his plug. If these women do not come with a set of built-in pathologies or psycho-social issues deep within their psyche (parental abuse, body shame, feelings of insecurity), then these Super Traits of these womens' temperaments are an even worthier mountain to summit.

The Super Traits, uncovered during the stalking and wooing phase, as Brown points out, prove the perfect complement to what the Psychopath brings to the relationship. She balances him out. He sees her the way Renee Zellwegger saw Tom Cruise in Jerry Maguire: she completes him. But only for so long. and only on his term.

Brown's Super Traits below do not cover, as Brown cautions, all of a woman's traits, but to a Psychopath, they tend to be the ones that are most highly elevated, the most highly prized. Here are the ones Brown has picked out as the most desired (and, as stated above, most of which just also happen to be the most cruelly ironic):

- **Extraversion and Excitement Seeking.** (Psychopaths are also extraverts and excitement seekers.) In other words, these women started out being the least dependent types on the planet!
- **Relationship Investment.** The victim gives great emotional, spiritual, physical, financial investments in any of her relationships, not just the intimate ones.

- Attachment. She has a deep bonding capacity.
- Competitiveness. She is not likely to be run out of relationships—she will stand her ground. Again, not the co-dependent type at all.
- Low Harm Avoidance. She doesn't expect to be hurt, sees others through who she is. In other words, not a person looking to recreate an abusive relationship of childhood. In fact, more often than not, these women were never exposed to abuse of any kid as children.
- Cooperation.
- Hyper-empathy. This can actually be genetic.
- Responsibility and Resourcefulness.

Any woman would be not only mentally and socially strong and secure if gifted with just several of these Super Traits, she would also be the last person anyone would expect to give in to the wiles of a Psychopath. Cooperative, resourceful, averse to self-abuse or abuse from others? And these are qualities that Psychopaths are attracted to? Qualities that seem to doom these Super Trait women to a pathological relationship? Unfortunately, for women who are not on their guard, who trust just a little too much, who possess an abundance of empathy, who are not at all codependent—Psychopaths relish the challenge of taking down a woman as accomplished and empowered as this. As Brown says: these traits are what many women have aspired toward and worked hard for over the past

50 years. They're way above the norm. How awful that being so successful on so many levels turns out to be an Achilles heel—the catnip and the way in for the Psychopath.

And yet many women with these Super Traits and more succumb to Psychopaths. How? Why? These women, like those of Morningstar's Just World, have just the right amount of compassion, just the right amount of a need for connection, a desire for romance and maybe too much of a sense of security. Put it all together and you have a woman who's just ripe as Psychopath's next casualty.

But in reality, it's not just women with these Super Traits who are put through these toxic relationships. There are plenty of women (and men) who go through the exact same abuse—the gaslighting, the lies, the hypnosis, the deception, the cajoling, the mind control. So why them? In short, taking Brown's theory but applying it to the Psychopaths as well, it makes just as much sense that there are Psychopaths out there who are not super-devious, who are not as accomplished, as experienced, as devious and manipulative as those Psychopaths who prey on these Super Trait women. And there are women out there who have no Super Traits, or who have just a few, or one or two. And so it would make absolute sense that, just as water seeks out its own level, there are these junior-league Psychopaths who seek out partners who are either as "level" as they are (as unsophisticated, as junior league, as average in their Psychopathology), or who will challenge them by being just a little above their Psychpathic pay grade—and so, just as much a challenge, just as much a triumph.

As if to prove this point, Brown relates a story about leading Psychopaths in a group therapy session some years ago. When she asked them how they chose their targets, they said it was pretty simple. They listened. Let a woman talk, let anyone talk, and they'll tell you everything you need to know about them— all their weak spots, all their deepest desires, where they're most vulnerable. And once they've overshared with you all of their secrets, all the things they're most wanting in life, out of life, you just spoon it back to them. And you're in.

Chapter 6: The Everyday Sadist

Such a brute should underneath all his braggart tricks, his viciousness, his vileness, be a coward. But I am convinced that he was not. Because even cowardice requires a certain degree of sensitivity, and a certain value for life.

Warren Eyster, *The Goblins of Eros*

The Everyday Sadist, now one of the Dark Traits (as part of the Dark Tetrad), and as is the case with the three other Dark Personalities, overlaps with the traits of Machiavellianism, Narcissism, and Psychopathy, but what they share most of all is callousness. Everyday Sadists, though, are not so much pathologically, clinically, or subclinically impulsive or manipulative as they are enjoyers of cruelty. They like to cause others pain, or they enjoy knowing or watching others suffer. And by pain, it's not just physical. In fact, Everyday Sadists will just as often bring the pain verbally (or via the internet or an electronic device) as physically.

Etymologically named after and forever unfortunately, and misleadingly, associated with the cruel sexual fetishes of the

French Revolutionary Era nobleman the Marquis de Sade, Sadism had a brief moment in the *Diagnostic and Statistical Manual of Mental Disorders.* In the now-defunct entry that once existed, Sadistic Personality Disorder back then was described as someone with an enduring and maladaptive pattern of dominating and abusing others with cruel, humiliating, or aggressive behavior. Although later removed from the *DSM* (due in part to political concerns that the definition may encourage male diagnostic bias and be used as a defense in domestic violence cases), Sadism as a diagnosis still carries weight among many clinical practitioners.

In their 2011 paper, "The Psychometric Properties and Utility of the Short Sadistic Impulse Scale (SSIS), applied psychologists Aisling O'Meara and Sean Hammond and clinical psychologist Jason Davies of Great Britain pointed out the dearth of studies on Sadism and the murkiness of what is available, characterizing the disorder as muddy and haphazardly diagnosed. Also, they rightly pointed out how Sadism is still lumped in with and seen as a purely sexual condition. Even the research done on Sadism seemed to focus unevenly, and unrewardingly, on sexual offenders, who didn't add any clarity to Sadism whatsoever.

Their solution? Give the field a clear and concise definition, which they did. Which others have since incorporated into their understanding of what Sadism is. Which boils down to anyone who has shown a long-term interest in cruel behavior to others, their pain, or the suffering of others for nothing more than their own pleasure.

As the co-originator of the term Dark Triad, Delroy Paulhus went one Dark Trait further in 2014, raising the case that the Everyday Sadist should be added to the Triad, and that the Dark Traits should henceforth be known as the Dark Tetrad. Although hard to make it official, most clinical practitioners and researchers seem to have accepted Paulhus' bid on behalf of the Everyday Sadist, especially as new studies continue to validate his argument on its pathological behalf.

Sadists All

It's a bit of a given that most if not all people have sadistic thoughts, or have a little bit of a sadist in them. This does not, obviously, qualify everyone as a sadist, or even a latent sadist (even when given the right opportunity—as proven by psychologist Philip Zimbardo in his 1971 Stanford prison experiment, in which Stanford undergraduates took part as prisoners and guard in a mock prison, and soon proved that people are only too easily persuaded to inflict pain on others, and others are only too eager to submit to such authoritarian cruelty. It has long been held that humans have an instinctual drive toward aggression and cruelty).

Nevertheless, humans aggress. Humans kill their own species—and often without reason or cause, and sometimes solely for pleasure. As far as cruelty goes, as it relates to Sadism, humans also appear to have a fascination with the spectacle of violence, either as participants or viewers. This fascination seems to transcend time and culture. Humans, not all but plenty, derive pleasure out of seeing others hurt. It could be argued that there's a potential Everyday Sadist lurking in all of us, but guilt, conscience, circumstance, context, whatever, keeps it tamped down. Or hidden.

If these collective conjectures are correct, then an appetitive motivation to inflict suffering may be present in all people, and the only difference between sadists and non-sadists is that the latter group has found a method to conquer their inner cruelty.

As to the Everyday Sadist, a sadistic personality can center on many things. The will, as some researchers have said, to disparage and humiliate, to exercise absolute power and unrestricted control over another, or the satisfaction derived from someone else's suffering. Sadists like to intentionally inflict physical, sexual, or psychological pain or suffering on others, strictly for their own pleasure.

The enjoyment of the sadistic act can come via direct participation (core sadism) or not so directly, such as watching others inflict pain and suffering (vicarious sadism). The late American psychologist Theodore Millon proposed four types of sadism: enforcing sadism, explosive sadism, spineless sadism, and tyrannical sadism. The Everyday Sadist might have the traits of one or all four of these types, though each of these subtypes tend to stay within their personality traits. According to Millon's definition, the Spineless Sadist is insecure, cowardly, tends to swagger and brag, and picks out powerless scapegoats as targets. The Tyrannical Sadist loves to menace and brutalize others, hoping for their submission, cuts people down verbally, is accusatory and destructive, and tends to be surly, abusive, and inhumane; in a word: a bully, whether in person or online (internet trolls are largely Tyrannical Sadists). The Enforcing Sadist are usually police officers, bossy supervisors, deans, judges, those who sublimate their hostility into the larger good, and therefore as public servants, profess the right to act harshly; they like to control and punish, and feel it their duty to ferret out rule breakers. The Explosive Sadist has a deep reservoir of bottled-up and often uncontrollable rage, and is prone to unpredictable and violent physical and verbal outbursts, only to later show contrition.

The Everyday Sadist can be any one of these Sadist subtypes. And true Sadists experience a kind of rush, repeatedly, whenever hurting others, and often, they lack the appropriate level of conscience needed to keep their addiction to sadistic pleasure under control.

Below are some of the more common outward traits of the typical Everyday Sadist.

They enjoy seeing people hurt and suffering. This could mean anything—from starting a rumor to publicly shaming someone, all just so they can watch that person squirm, and know that they caused that person their pain.

They enjoy hurting people. They enjoy bringing physical harm and pain to others. For example, this particular Sadist is standing in line at the movies. They don't like that the person behind them is standing too close, so they accidentally stomp on that person's foot.

They get excited by the idea of knowing others are in pain. A fight breaks out on the sidewalk. The Sadist doesn't shy away or call for help. They're right there, glued to the action. The violence, especially the suddenness of it, appeals to them.

They think it is acceptable to cause others' pain. Taking a kind of nihilistic, Hobbesian do or be done to approach to life, Sadists espouse a kind of affectless acceptance of kill or be killed. Hurt others before, or lest, they hurt you. Either way, they're OK with it.

They fantasize about hurting others. Sadists can drift off to thoughts of torture, mayhem, revenge fantasies, cruel sexual fantasies—all with a smile on their face.

They hurt others because they can. Squashing bugs seems OK. But when it's just for pleasure—that's sadistic. Similarly, Sadists think it's OK to bully others, and lately, they think it's especially OK to do it anonymously, online, where there are almost no consequences.

They like being humiliating others in order to keep them in line. If you're engaged in an argument with a Sadist, don't be surprised if they go from their inside voice to their outside voice in seconds—all the better to draw the attention of others and put you into an uncomfortable, embarrassing position.

Their sexual tendencies have an edge to them. If they want you to submit to sexual acts such as bondage, gagging, slapping, hair pulling, choking.

Sadism! It's Not Just for Sexual Deviants and Criminals Anymore

In their July 2017 paper, "Everyday sadism, the Dark Triad, personality, and disgust sensitivity," Myrthe Meere and

Vincent Egan stated that exraversion (someone who's the life of the party), Psychopathy, Machiavellianism, and animal reminder disgust (the idea that we humans have evolved to be disgusted by any reminder that we are animals) were significant predictors of **S**adism scores.

In 2012, University of British Columbia grad student Erin Evelyn Buckels published a paper, written for her MA and titled *The Pleasures of Hurting Others: Behavioral Evidence of Everyday Sadism*. In it, she detailed two studies, one of which revealed that people who score high on a measure of sadism don't mind going that extra mile if it means making someone else suffer. Disturbing?

Buckels seems intent on establishing a less emotional approach to Sadism and Sadists. Even people most of us would consider fine, upstanding citizens can get off watching someone else suffer (Saw didn't become a box-office smash and produce eight sequels—and counting—because we're a nation of bunny lovers. And just because these people have a predilection for other people's pain, be it vicariously or personally inflicted, does not mean they're all serial murderers or sexual predators. There's an emotional need being scratched here. And Buckels, and more and more other researchers, want to know why. And what this Dark Psychology, this Dark Trait might say about individuals, about society.

Buckels later teamed up with Delroy Paulhus (and Daniel Jones of the University of El Paso), and with them published her two MA studies. In combination with Paulhus' previous work on the Dark Triad (now Tetrad), the three concluded that sadists possess an intrinsic motivation to inflict suffering on innocent others, even at a personal cost — a motivation that is absent from the other dark personality traits.

The researchers hope that these new findings will help to broaden people's view of sadism as an aspect of personality that manifests in everyday life, helping to dispel the notion that sadism is limited to sexual deviants and criminals.

Sadists Online and on Social Media

Other areas of interest to clinical psychologists and Dark Psychology researchers are social media and the internet. Sadists and Psychopaths seem drawn to websites like Facebook and media like Twitter—more so than the other Dark Personalities. And their activities of choice seems to be cyberstalking, cyberbullying, and trolling.

Various studies have confirmed that trolls exhibit traits partial to Sadists, at least a little, as Buckels and Paulhus and others concluded in a 2018 study, "Internet trolling and everyday sadism: Parallel effects on pain perception and moral judgment." Trolls are different, for sure. If for no other reason than that they seem, to Buckels, to lean toward the Sadistic.

And if we are all potential trolls, as Christian Jarrett believes, then that only bolsters the argument that we are all also potential Sadists.

Twitter seems to bring out the worst in our nature, partly due to the online disinhibition effect, partly due to the anonymity of smartphones and the internet, all of which heighten the propensity to behave irresponsibly if not immorally. And research has suggested that people already susceptible to their inner Everyday Sadist have a high tendency to troll others online; while Buckels and Paulhus' 2018 study showed that being in a bad mood and going onto social media and then exposing oneself to trolls, doubles the likelihood that that person will themselves then in turn troll others, creating a vicious cycle of spiteful, sadistic trolling.

Chapter 7: Dark Techniques

Men are so simple of mind, and so much dominated by their immediate needs, that a deceitful man will always find plenty who are ready to be deceived.

Niccoló Machiavelli, *The Prince*

Dark methods, dark modes, dark systems, dark tactics. Dark Psychology largely boils down to people who are practicing, consciously and/or unconsciously, manipulation and mind control. It is that simple. To those two can also be added a laundry list of other practices and techniques: brainwashing, lying, deception, delusion, gaslighting, NeuroLinguistic Programming, social conditioning, social engineering, reverse engineering, influence, dominate, master to the above, and you've pretty much covered the Dark Techniques. And while these are all variations on essentially the same thing, varying only slightly in how they're each done, their goals are but one: control. Control over others. (Some might add power, but one cannot attain or maintain power without first having control—first over oneself, then over others.)

Again, it's that simple.

And keep in mind: These are Dark Techniques. If you're dealing with a Narcissist, a Psychopath, an Everyday Sadist, a Machiavellian—the more you know about their methods, the better you'll be able to deal with them. Or keep your distance from them. Not all of them are evil, or sinister. Everyone most likely employs one or more or all of them at some point in their lives. Or uses them on a daily basis. Manipulation, coercion, persuasion—maybe you're in marketing or advertising. You use these techniques every day. It's your business. The difference here, with all these techniques, is intent. Are you wanting to win over a client or your supervisor and not sure the best way to do that? Certainly, there's something to be learned, something of value, something probably of use here in the Dark Techniques. Are you wanting to hone your skills of seduction and attract more women—or the right kind of woman for you? Same thing. There are techniques here that, though well within the skill set of a Psychopath they're useful to everyone. And used by everyone. Psychopaths don't have a copyright on any of these techniques. Nor should you feel that it's not your right to try out some of these techniques. Again, it comes down to intent—with great power comes great responsibility.

Certainly, then, there are positives to be found in Dark Psychology. If only to know who these Dark Types are and how they move through the world. As Sun Tzu put it almost 2,500 years ago: "If you know the enemy and know yourself, you need not fear the result of a hundred battles. If you know yourself but not the enemy, for every victory gained you will also suffer a defeat. If you know neither the enemy nor yourself, you will succumb in every battle."

The danger lies in not emulating these Dark actors too too much. Or with ill intent. As Ernest O'Boyle, associate professor of management at the Kelley School of Business at Indiana University observed in a story for Science that asked "Does a 'Dark Triad' of personality traits make you more successful?", there's the possibility of going too far, of investing too much time and energy into these Dark Traits and Dark Personality types. As Friedrich Nietzsche cautioned long ago, "Whoever fights *monsters* should see to it that in the process he does not become a *monster*. And if you gaze long enough into an abyss, the abyss will gaze back into you."

Chapter 8: Manipulation

Dark Psychology is all about manipulation. That's its essence. Every Dark Personality, every Dark Trait, almost every Dark Tactic has at its root manipulation.

Manipulation is all around us—through advertising, marketing, from our parents, our supervisors, our lovers, the layout of our local mall. It so completely is a part of our lives we hardly notice it. So when a Psychopath, a Machiavellian approaches us with a request, an ask, a piece of information, no wonder we're not always aware that they're after something. Us, most likely. Or something we have—money, power, our bodies. And we all do it, sometimes it's just a white lie, sometimes flattery, sometimes complete subterfuge. For those of the Dark Triad, however, manipulation is a way of life. They are, to be ungentle about it, predators. And we are their prey.

But let's also be clear about the difference between manipulation and influence. (Influence, it could be argued— that's really what's all around us, via ads and the internet and from our friends and teachers. And subliminal influencing, via subliminal messages, those are definitely covert and underhanded, but used less by individual Dark Personalities and more by governments, advertising, TV, music, and movies—as popularized and demonized in Vance Packard's 1957 classic expose, *The Hidden Persuaders*, in which Packard claimed that advertisers were manipulating Americans' unconscious desires so that they'd buy products they didn't need. Manipulative, for sure. Pathological, no.)

So. The Difference between manipulation and influence. Manipulation often causes confusion, anxiety, depression, and powerlessness. It's unpleasant, it's demeaning. Manipulative relationships are destructive. Manipulators do not care what happens to their targets. Manipulators only want what they want—and the consequences be damned.

People who seek to influence others, they have a positive intent. Their self-esteem does not depend on the actions of the person they are seeking to influence. Influence also involves open and direct communication. The influencer behaves with clarity and transparency and a clear goal, which is usually to the benefit of both parties, if not entirely for the benefit of the person being influenced. And the person being influenced is not just allowed to think for themselves, they're often encouraged think for themselves and to make their own decisions.

Manipulators lie. They manipulate covertly, indirectly, underhandedly. They feel justified, entitled, *rightful* to treat others however they choose. Manipulators also see the world in zero-sum terms. Play or get played. Eat or be eaten. The world to them is black and white. For them, a relationship is a power struggle, a connection but one on unequal terms. Terms in their favor, terms they control. Ultimately, they do not trust others—because they know that they themselves are not trustworthy.

Before I begin my attack, I must first become acquainted with her and her whole mental state.

Søren Kierkegaard, *The Seducer's Diary*

What sort of targets, then, do Manipulators prey on? Do they have a particular type? They do: someone with issues. Unresolved issues. Issues Manipulators can sniff out, then exploit. People with low self-esteem, who are naïve, easy to please, too eager to please, unassertive, lacking in confidence—these are the most vulnerable. People with certain weaknesses like the ones below. If any of these strike a chord, if you have any of these tendencies, any of these behaviors, work on them. Don't try to hide them or hope a Manipulator won't detect them. Work on them. They are:

An unhealthy need to please: The target, fearful of rejection, disapproval, abandonment—of introducing the slightest dose of reality into the relationship—keeps everything as pleasant as possible. (AKA the "disease to please.")

The need to earn the approval and acceptance of others: Sometimes corresponds to a lack of confidence in one's own judgments—especially of others. Especially when it comes to Manipulators—who put on a very convincing front but to a target, often just feel off. But without a solid sense of self, the target yields to others. This need for approval can then cloud one's trust in oneself, in one's visceral reaction to a Manipulator.

Cannot say No!: Or just No, thank you. A lack of assertiveness, especially, again, when it comes to one's feelings or one's own needs or wants.

Soft personal boundaries: A murky sense of who you are. Your identity rests too much in others and you tend to merge or lose yourself in another person's boundaries. A person just one step up from soft, who has spongy boundaries is, according to Old Dominion professor Nina Brown, author of *Coping With Infuriating, Mean, Critical People—The Destructive Narcissistic Pattern,* someone with soft and rigid boundaries. People with spongy boundaries are unsure of who to let in and who to keep out

Low self-reliance: You tend to cling to others and rely on them and can even see them as superior or more powerful. You're emotionally dependent, submissive.

A fear of negative emotions: You cannot express anger, frustration, or disapproval. What Harriet B. Braiker, author of *The Disease To Please*, calls "emotophobia."

The feeling that you don't feel in control and that everything is someone else's fault: If a locus of control is the degree to which people believe they have control over the outcome of events in their lives, people with an external locus of control blame (or thank) outside factors for what happens in their lives.

And two others: **the overly conscientious**—targets who are too willing to give a Manipulator the benefit of the doubt—and **the over-intellectualizer**—the target who is intent on figuring out why it is the Manipulator continues to do the things they do, all the while staying with the Manipulator rather than leaving.

Whether or not you are on this list, being manipulated is not your fault. Manipulators know what they're doing. They are in control. The manipulated, though, until they see it, they have little idea what's going on. Even so, it is still up to the target of the Manipulator to put up boundaries. That is not victim blaming, it's just how it is. The Manipulator will not stop until their target puts a stop to their behavior. Otherwise, there's no incentive. Things are working out great for them; they're getting exactly what they want. Why stop? The solution: Stop rewarding their tactics. Manipulation exists because it works.

The techniques of manipulation are many—and seemingly endless. Here are some—some of the ones used most often by Dark Personality types.

Love Bombing (aka **Love Flooding**): Unlike the display of a healthy romantic level of interest, Love Bombing happens too fast and comes on way too strong. The Manipulator immediately want to spend every moment with you; they're madly in love with you right there at the bar, in the middle of happy hour. According to Michael Pace, author of *Dark Psychology 101: Learn The Secrets Of Covert Emotional Manipulation, Dark Persuasion, Undetected Mind Control, Mind Games, Deception, Hypnotism, Brainwashing And Other Tricks Of The Trade*, Love bombing has almost nothing to do with love. It's all a ruse—the early stage of the Manipulator readying his victim.

Positive Reinforcement: After the Love Bombing comes positive reinforcement, which comes in many forms, from outright praise and superficial charm to superficial sympathy (crocodile tears) and excessive apologizing. As *Dark Psychology* author Michael Pace explains it, this comes soon after the Love Bombing. Only it's hardly at all positive. Instead, the Manipulator has stopped Love Bombing altogether and replaced it with . . . crickets. For instance, the target must wear a certain dress the Manipulator gave them before the Manipulator will give them a kiss. The target has no idea that the kiss comes not from the Manipulator's desire for her, it's because he coerced her into doing what he wanted.

Negative Reinforcement: To give you an idea of why Manipulators love this tactic, it was championed by American psychologist B.F. Skinner, whose philosophy was "radical behaviorism." Skinner also suggested that the concept of free will was simply an illusion, and believed that all human action was the direct result of conditioning. Negative reinforcement is a response or behavior that's strengthened by stopping, removing, or avoiding a negative outcome or aversive stimulus. You decide to stop crying because of your menstrual cramps (behavior) in order to avoid getting into a fight over your crying (removal of the aversive stimulus). Even though that behavior is not deliberate, the Manipulator uses negative reinforcement to get you, the target, to adopt to his wishes, his demands—no matter how unreasonable.

Love Denial/Love Withdrawal: First he Giveth, then he Taketh away. After all that love, the Manipulator lets the target know just who's boss by withdrawing all that love and attention and affection. If the Manipulator doesn't out-and-out leave, their love—its quality, its frequency, its expression—

morphs into something altogether . . . different. As if you have less value than the day before they professed their undying love for you.

Lying: Manipulators lie. They tell half-truths. They misinform, disinform, mislead, and exaggerate. (See Lying, below, for more about this tactic.)

Not Telling the Whole Story: Distinct from outright Lying, the Manipulator withholds a key piece of information, the key part of the story, in order to keep their target at a disadvantage.

Denial: "I never said that." "I never did that." When the Manipulator refuses to admit they said or did something wrong, offensive, or hurtful.

Rationalization: A defense mechanism in which the Manipulator makes an excuse for inappropriate behavior. As the *DSM* defines it, it's when the individual deals with emotional conflict or internal or external stressors by concealing the true motivations for his or her own thoughts, actions, or feelings through the elaboration of reassuring or self-serving but incorrect explanations. Also known as spin.

Minimization: Denial + Rationalization = Minimization. When the Manipulator defends their actions, or something they said, usually a sarcastic taunt or insult, with the excuse that "It was only a joke." (Sarcasm as a reaction is benign. Sarcasm from a Manipulator has a demeaning, passive-aggressive purpose to it.) Playing down their actions as not important or damaging, thereby shifting the blame onto the target for overreacting.

Passive-Aggressiveness: A form of avoidance where the Manipulator, often by procrastinating, pouting, being stubborn, withholding sex, silent treatment, acts that are indirectly aggressive rather than directly aggressive, all the while wanting a specific response.

Leading Questions: Questions that set you up for the kill. In a normal relationship, one partner asks the other, How's our relationship going? In a manipulative relationship, the Manipulator asks, Were you making out with Nick behind the gym last night? These questions have an implied or explicit answer or assumption. It's the opposite of empathic listening—and designed as a set-up for the target, i.e., no matter how the target answers, they lose.

Mood Swings: The Manipulator, being ever unpredictable as to who the target will be dealing with when the Manipulator returns home, keeps the target forever off-balance and walking on eggshells.

Guilt Trips: Another passive-aggressive ploy, intended to make the target feel "less than." Example: If you'd only done what I'd asked you to do, we wouldn't be stuck here having this conversation. Or, You don't care enough. You're so selfish. You have it so easy. This leaves the target feeling bad, in self-doubt, anxious, and/or submissive.

Reverse Psychology: Subtly encouraging a belief or a behavior by upholding its opposite.

Mind Games: Another passive-aggressive ploy of one-upmanship designed to disemploy and disempower the target while further empowering the Manipulator. AKA Mind Fucks, Head Games, and Power Games. Often rely on social embarrassment and Semantic Manipulation (see below).

Punishment: Nagging (constant), shouting (often, unpredictable), the silent treatment, withholding sex. Applied randomly by the Manipulator, with the target not knowing what they did wrong.

Semantic Manipulation: A communication tactic that sidesteps a problem or an issue by manipulating the target into accepting something, or doing something, they otherwise would not accept or do. Often deployed in the midst of a compromise or negotiation (T—I asked to have the house to myself on Sundays, not Tuesdays. I work Tuesdays. M—No, you specifically told me Tuesdays because you said you were gonna change your hours.)

Selective Attention/Inattention: This is when the Manipulator refuses to pay attention to whatever may interfere with their desires, their agenda. For example: "I don't want to hear it." End of discussion.

Isolation: Knowing that it is far easier to keep a person under control if they are isolated from family members and friends who could shed some light and truth on the situation, the Manipulator transitions from "Let's just you and me stay home tonight" to "I don't really like your friends and family. I just like being with you."

Diversion: The Manipulator can't give you a straight answer, not even to a Yes or No question, and instead steers the conversation to another topic.

Evasion: Like Diversion but the Manipulator gives vague, rambling, irrelevant responses—weasel words—words or statements that are intentionally misleading or ambiguous.

Shaming: The Manipulator uses sarcasm and put-downs to increase fear and self-doubt in the target. Shaming can be very subtle—a disappointed look, a mean glance, a tone of voice—and are hugely effective at fostering a sense of inadequacy in the target.

Vilifying the Victim: Often used by the Manipulator as a way to alleviate their guilt over a wrongdoing they've committed, this is when the Manipulator depicts someone else in the worst possible light in order to justify their own behaviors. It's a rather ingenious way of creating confusion about who the real target is. They falsely blame others to shirk free of any responsibility or accountability for their actions. I slept with your best friend but you pushed me into it. It puts the victim (the target) on the defensive while simultaneously masking the aggressive intent of the Manipulator (they did something hurtful). Worse, if the target defends themselves or their position, the Manipulator, in response, falsely accuses the target as being the abuser.

Playing the Victim: The Manipulator portrays himself as a victim of circumstance or of someone else's behavior in order to gain pity, sympathy or evoke compassion and thereby get something from another.

Playing the Servant: Cloaking a self-serving agenda in a noble cause. Manipulator: I have to fill in for the owner this weekend, so you'll have to deal with the kids on your own.

Projecting Blame (Blaming Others): Manipulators are so effective because unless they work in such subtle, hard-to-detect, nearly impossible to explain ways. Projecting blame, where the Manipulator scapegoats the target, is particularly insidious. A combination of misdirection and blame-shifting, the Manipulator casts their flaws and feelings onto the target:

"I was late for an important meeting because you said I had to pick up the kids." Projecting blame is frequently used as a means of psychological and emotional manipulation and control. Manipulators lie about lying, only to re-manipulate the original, less believable story into a "more acceptable" truth that the target will believe. Projecting lies as being the truth is another common tactic. Manipulators love to falsely accuse the target as "deserving to be treated that way." They often claim that the target is crazy and/or abusive, especially when there is evidence against the Manipulator. (See Feigning, below.)

Moving the Goalposts: You might think you know where you stand with a Manipulator, but if they are constantly moving the goalposts in order to confuse you, then it's likely you're dealing with a predator. The ground is always shifting. One day the Manipulator tells you to leave the lights on, the next day he berates you for not having turned the lights off.

Gaslighting: A nefarious tactic, akin to brainwashing. The Manipulator causes the target to doubt herself, and ultimately lose her own sense of perception, identity, and self-worth. Derived from the 1944 film *Gaslight,* in which a Charles Boyer's character tries to convince his wife, Ingrid Bergman, that she's insane. Bergman keeps seeing gaslights (19th-century lamps) dimming and brightening for no apparent reason. Boyer convinces her it's all inside her head. In reality, he was switching the attic lights on and off to create the gaslight flickers. The Manipulator: C'mon. I never told you that. Or: You're being paranoid. Or: Why are you making such a big deal out of this?

Feigning Innocence/Ignorance: The Manipulator, playing the innocence card, tries to suggest that any harm done was unintentional or they did not do something that they were accused of. The target feels like a false accuser, a perpetrator, and often questions their own judgment and possibly their own sanity.

Feigning Confusion: The Manipulator plays dumb, pretending they do not know what the target is talking about or they're confused about an important issue brought to their attention. The Manipulator intentionally confuses the target in order for the target to doubt their own accuracy of perception, often pointing out key elements that the Manipulator intentionally included in case there is room for doubt.

Brandishing Anger: The Manipulator uses anger, emotional intensity, and rage to shock the target into submission. The Manipulator is not actually angry, it's just an act. The "anger" is also effective as a way for the Manipulator to avoid telling truths at inconvenient times or circumstances; the target— scared, uncertain if the anger is genuine or not—becomes more focused on the anger instead of either the original topic or the manipulation tactic.

Bandwagon Effect: The Manipulator comforts the target into submission by claiming (whether true or false) that other people are doing it, so you can too. It often occurs in scenarios where the Manipulator tries to influence the target into trying drugs or sexual acts.

If any of these scenarios or behaviors hits a nerve, there's manipulation going on. And the only real way to stop the manipulation from continuing is to stop falling into the manipulation. Don't fool yourself into thinking that if the Manipulator knew better they would treat you better. The more victimized you feel, the less you will feel able to powerful over yourself or your life. As you become more diminished, you become more vulnerable to manipulation in the future. So don't try to change the manipulator, focus on changing you and your behavior.

Chapter 9: Brainwashing/Mind Control

The most dramatic instances of directed behavior change and "mind control" are not the consequence of exotic forms of influence, such as hypnosis, psychotropic drugs, or "brainwashing," but rather the systematic manipulation of the most mundane aspects of human nature over time in confining settings.

Philip Zimbardo, author of *The Lucifer Effect: Understanding How Good People Turn Evil* and conductor of the 1971 Stanford prison experiment

Brainwashing, as Lisa Aronson Fontes, a psychology researcher at the University of Massachusetts Amherst and author of *Invisible Chains: Overcoming Coercive Control in Your Intimate Relationship*, told *Business Insider* in 2017, basically means not having the wherewithal, the confidence, to know yourself or the world outside you. First appearing in the literature on the brainwashing of prisoners of war (think of the

1962 film *The Manchurian Candidate*), it has also been applied to people in cults, and has lately caught on in the world of Dark Psychology.

Not yet a scientific fact yet it made the *DSM-5*, brainwashing (or mind control) is the idea that you can persuade someone to do exactly what you want them to do. Better yet, you can get them to do things without them having the slightest idea you're doing it. Also known as Covert Emotional Manipulation, re-education, menticide, thought control, and thought reform, it came about in the 1950s as a way to try to explain how China's government got so many people to cooperate with its policies.

Then, in 1957, U.S. Air Force sociologist Albert Biderman published a report that studied how Chinese Communist interrogators managed to pull military intelligence out of U.S. prisoners interned at a war camp during the Korean War. The American prisoners gave up tactical information, collaborated with Chinese propaganda, and signed on to false confessions. In his report, Biderman stated that inflicting physical pain was not necessary to get the prisoners to do what they were told, as the interrogators' psychological methods of coercion proved more than effective. His report also outlined what came to be known as "Biderman's Chart of Coercion," in which Biderman delineated the mechanisms for brainwashing:

- Isolation

- Monopolization of perception (fixes attention on immediate predicament; eliminates "undesirable" stimuli)
- Induced debilitation; exhaustion
- Threats
- Occasional indulgences (provides motivation for compliance; hinders adjustment to deprivation)
- Demonstrating superiority
- Degradation
- Enforcing trivial demands

Interpersonally, within relationships, Psychopaths, Everyday Sadists, and even Narcissists have come to employ many of these same mind control techniques, victimizing their partners through what Fontes calls "perspecticide." Perspecticide sets in when the abuser convinces the victim of so many things that aren't true that the victim no longer has any idea what is real and what is not. The victim essentially becomes a prisoner in their own life—unable to think or do anything stemming from their own will.

People who set out to brainwash others, like any Manipulator, their best candidates for mind control are people with a hole inside. They're missing something—self-esteem, self-confidence, a father figure. It's something they crave. Almost like an addict in search of that initial high.

It's the kind of craving that cult leaders and Psychopaths, military recruiters and Narcissists, terrorist cells and sexual slavery rings prey on. In his 1961 book *Thought Reform and the Psychology of Totalism: A Study of "Brainwashing" in China*, psychiatrist Robert Jay Lifton, an authority on cults and brainwashing, set down the "Eight Criteria for Thought Reform." These criteria are almost identical to the techniques applied by your everyday Manipulator. It's only a difference, really, of scale. Lifton came up with these tactics more in relation to a group dynamic than a one-on-one relationship. Milieu Control, in which the victim is cut off from the outside world physically and psychologically, is pretty much the same as Isolation. Loading the Language, where the group interprets or uses words and phrases in new ways and in such a particular way is no different from the way the Seducer (see below) should wield their words in ways that discombobulate and distract the Seduced. And Dispensing of Existence, where only the group decides who exists and who does not—is this not the essence, the endgame, of the Manipulator?

In brainwashing, the one doing the washing empties out the mind of the follower and puts into it whatever he feels is right and appropriate. He tells the brainwashed who they now are, what was wrong with them, how they need to change. The brainwashed has been cleaned out of past memories, past feelings, past thoughts. And reprogrammed.

Chapter 10: Seduction

It is not enough to conquer; one must learn to seduce.

Voltaire

Seduction via Dark Psychology is not to be trifled with. If you are intent on seducing someone using the methods of the Narcissist, the Machiavellian, the Psychopath—what is your intent? Do you fancy yourself as dark as these subclinical pathological types? Or are you merely wanting to learn from them—pick up a trick of the trade that might make it easier to meet someone, to maintain a relationship? Or is your goal to see things from the inside so that you're less susceptible to a Dark Seducer?

As Julien Fabrice, creator of the blog Diary of a French PUA (PUA being the acronym for Pick-Up Artist, a person who practices finding, attracting, and seducing sexual partners). Explaining how and why he set up his own PUA blog, he sees his sharing of his exploits as a public service. He's giving a leg up to all the Joe Schmoes out there, the ones with less confidence, less (self) awareness. He's showing them the tricks of the Manipulator's trade. This is how the alpha dogs, the top seducers, do it. And once I've showed you what's behind the curtain, you'll be that much harder to fool. You'll be in on the game instead of standing outside, wondering how all these other guys that look just like him have managed to sweet talk that hot chick into bed. Because an alpha, supposedly, is not a sucker that is easily manipulated." Fabrice is part of a very loose PUA community, mostly of men, a community that keeps in touch via chat rooms, internet newsletters, blogs, forums, and clubs around the world (known as "lairs").

Seduction is all about manipulation. And the language, the words used when talking about seduction, or writing about it— many of them have to do not only with magic and deception, illusion and fantasy, but are the exact same concepts, terminologies, and techniques that show up in Narcissism, Machiavellianism, Psychopathy, and Everyday Sadism. Women are prey. Seducers have few morals. They keep you on eggshells (if admittedly less stressful more sexy eggshells, they're still eggshells). They lull you into a false sense of security. Sound familiar? Sound like everything that's in the Dark Triad's bag of evil tricks? You bet it does. It's just that the intent, maybe, is a little less evil, a little less venal.

By now it should be clear, especially in this chapter on seduction, that in any book or blog or article or YouTube tutorial that's giving you advice on how to pick up chicks, how to seduce, how to get someone to do what you want them to do—which is really what Dark Psychology, what psychology, period (in a way), ultimately boils down to—is all about, especially when that someone is you. After all, you're really just trying to teach yourself, push yourself, trick yourself, into doing what you want YOU to do. Not someone else, you.

It's rarely stated so nakedly, but that's really the goal. Even if it's just a side benefit, it's still valuable. It will still help you.

As one writer admits, the benefit of sitting down with Robert Greene's massive but entertainingly cerebral self-help book *The Art of Seduction*, aside from being fun, aside from having a lot of great stories and decent "advice," the hidden benefit of reading it is coming away with a better idea of how not to be the victim. Sure, you may follow through on some of Greene's moves, but the real pleasure, the true satisfaction comes more in being able to spot a seducer, spot a victim. We're all seducers and victims at some point in our lives. Which is also the point of Dark Psychology and Dark Traits, and the crossover among them, and the fluidity. We are not all one thing. We are rarely, few of us, are always just guided by the behaviors of a Psychopath, or a Narcissist. Hell, even Hitler is said to have loved dogs. Hitler, the most loathsome sociopathic Narcissist in history (or one of the most loathsome). And one of the Master Seducers of all time. He had other qualities. Imagine. Some of them even halfway decent. Qualities and behaviors that if we came across them in the little old lady down the street we'd shed a tear over. But because it's Hitler, we somehow can't see him as anything but pure evil. As the essence of Dark Psychology. Dark Psychology taken to its most unimaginable extreme.

Yet we can learn from him. And from other Machiavellians and Psychopaths as well. (Obviously, though, you don't want to go around bragging about how you learned this really effective seduction technique based on something Hitler, or Himmler, or Mussolini used.)

So. Seduction. As Fabrice, the PUA, said, part of the takeaway of his own writings, part of the takeaway of this e-book, is for you to be less susceptible to mind control, to seducers, to brainwashing. To the worst of the Tribe of the Dark Traits. If seduction is all about power and control, and knowledge is power, then having more knowledge, a keener insight, of those who are out there vying for power and control, trying to control others, trying to control *you*, well, you'll move through the world a little more comfortably, a little more confidently. That's not to say you won't be immune to the Dark Trait Tribe, but you should be able to spot them more quickly, and decide for yourself whether or not you want them in your life, and if so, to what degree.

Again. Seduction. Seduction we've already covered in the previous chapters—that's what the Psychopaths do, the

Narcissists, the Machiavellians, the Everyday Sadists. They just had darker intentions. If you take some of their techniques from above and rejigger them as Seduction—maybe as techniques in the Art of Romantic Seduction, you'll do fine. In fact, you'll probably do more than fine.

As Greene himself points out in *The Art of Seduction*, the origin of the word seduction is to "lead astray." By now, you should have a better idea of how others have been trying to seduce you, trying to lead you astray, down a path that they chose, not that you chose. Choose your own path. Seduce yourself first. Then decide who you want to seduce next.

Chapter 11: The Dark End

In closing, Dark Psychology is still in its infancy in terms of studying it and learning from it—and learning from the people, the Dark Personalities, who live there. It's not a fun place, but as Delroy Paulhus seems to feel, hanging out with a Psychopath or a Machiavellian would certainly be more interesting and maybe even more fun at times than spending the weekend with an agoraphobic.

And make no mistakes, these Dark Triad/Tetrad characters, they've been with us since we were upright. They may be dangerous at times, and wreak havoc and cause damage, but they also contribute to whatever society they're a part of. And they're a part of every society. And contributing to a society's well-being, not just to its darker sides.

Take Dan Mallory, for instance. He's the best-selling author of the debut thriller, *The Woman in the Window*. Bright, young, talented, successful—and very likely a Psychopath. In a *New Yorker* profile from February 2019 titled "Unreliable Narrator," coworkers describe him in Dark terms. Not *dark* Dark. But dark enough, disturbing enough, questionable enough, that it earned him more of an expose than a profile in a major American magazine. Psychopathic. Guilty of gaslighting. Narcissistic. Dark enough that he could easily serve as a textbook case in the annals of Dark Psychology.

If there's any doubt that these Dark Personalities are out there, among us, in the public eye, even serving as role models of sorts, Mallory's presence, and popularity, shows just how maddening, and maddeningly fascinating, these Dark Personality types can be. And how they still have plenty to teach us—about ourselves, about what makes people tick, what makes them behave the way do, what makes them think they can behave so darkly. And get away with it. Which they often do.

Made in the USA
Las Vegas, NV
28 June 2021